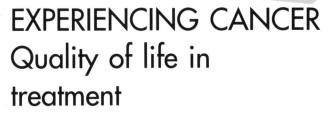

EXPERIENCING CANCER
Quality of life in treatment

KIRSTEN COSTAIN SCHOU
JENNY HEWISON

OPEN UNIVERSITY PRESS
Buckingham · Philadelphia

Open University Press
Celtic Court
22 Ballmoor
Buckingham
MK18 1XW

email: enquiries@openup.co.uk
world wide web: http://www.openup.co.uk

and
325 Chestnut Street
Philadelphia, PA 19106, USA

First Published 1999

A catalogue record of this book is available from the British Library

ISBN 0 335 19892 9 (hb)   0 335 19891 0 (pb)

Library of Congress Cataloging-in-Publication Data
Schou, Kirsten Costain, 1964–
    Experiencing cancer : quality of life in treatment / Kirsten
Costain Schou and Jenny Hewison.
        p.   cm. — (Facing death)
    Includes bibliographical references and index.
    ISBN 0–335–19892–9 (hbk)   ISBN 0–335–19891–0 (pbk)
    1. Cancer—Patients—Care—Social aspects.   2. Quality of life—
Social aspects.   I. Hewison, Jenny, 1950– .   II. Title.
III. Series.
    [DNLM: 1. Neoplasms—therapy.   2. Neoplasms—psychology.
3. Quality of Life.   QZ 266 S376e 1998]
RC262.S435   1998
362.1'96994—dc21
DNLM/DLC
for Library of Congress

Typeset by Graphicraft Limited, Hong Kong
Printed in Great Britain by St Edmundsbury Press,
Bury St Edmunds, Suffolk

EXPERIENCING CANCER

FACING DEATH

Series editor: David Clark, Professor of Medical Sociology,
University of Sheffield

The subject of death in late modern culture has become a rich field of theoretical, clinical and policy interest. Widely regarded as a taboo until recent times, death now engages a growing interest among social scientists, practitioners and those responsible for the organization and delivery of human services. Indeed, how we die has become a powerful commentary on how we live and the specialized care of dying people holds an important place within modern health and social care.

This series captures such developments in a collection of volumes which has much to say about death, dying, end-of-life care and bereavement in contemporary society. Among the contributors are leading experts in death studies, from sociology, anthropology, social psychology, ethics, nursing, medicine and pastoral care. A particular feature of the series is its attention to the developing field of palliative care, viewed from the perspectives of practitioners, planners and policy analysts; here several authors adopt a multi-disciplinary approach, drawing on recent research, policy and organizational commentary, and reviews of evidence-based practice. Written in a clear, accessible style, the entire series will be essential reading for students of death, dying and bereavement and for anyone with an involvement in palliative care research, service delivery or policy making.

Current and forthcoming titles:

David Clark, Jo Hockley, Sam Ahmedzai (eds): *New Themes in Palliative Care*
David Clark and Jane Seymour: *Reflections on Palliative Care*
Mark Cobb: *Spiritual Issues in Palliative Care*
Kirsten Costain Schou and Jenny Hewison: *Experiencing Cancer: Quality of Life in Treatment*
David Field, David Clark, Jessica Corner and Carol Davis (eds): *Researching Palliative Care*
David Kissane and Sidney Bloch: *Family Grief Therapy*
Gordon Riches and Pamela Dawson: *An Intimate Loneliness: Supporting Bereaved Parents and Siblings*
Tony Walter: *On Bereavement*

Contents

Series editor's preface

At a time when there is much discussion about how the quality of cancer services can be improved (CMOEAG 1995) and how palliative care can become more integrated with oncology (Richards 1997), Kirsten Costain Schou and Jenny Hewison have produced an important book. For here is a work which provides an unusually detailed insight into the experience of cancer, from diagnosis through treatment and care. It is a story told in the words of people with cancer themselves, drawing on carefully conducted qualitative research. The authors use the novel concept of viewing cancer treatment as a series of 'calendars' – to be interpreted, negotiated and managed, by patients and also by health professionals. Within the calendar we are shown a number of complex processes and phases. These include diagnosis; prognostic assessment; surgery; radiotherapy; chemotherapy; and, follow-up. In each case detailed interview data provides startling insights into how these are perceived and experienced by people with cancer. This can make for riveting reading. It also reveals some of the insensitivities, misunderstandings and unfairnesses which may creep into a system concerned to provide high technology modern medicine, at speed, to those with a life-threatening malignant disease. We learn of the frustrations, the hopes, the aspirations associated with treatment. We encounter the mundane processes of travelling to and from the treatment centre and the sense of identification with fellow patients. We also come to understand the narratives which individuals use to make sense of their experience of cancer. There is a strong sense of embodiment about these accounts and we learn of the physicality of the illness, its ability to transform experiences of the body, and the bodily metaphors which are used to explain it.

This material should be essential reading for anyone interested in current developments in the sociology and social psychology of the body. It should also be read by those responsible for planning and delivering cancer services. For here we get beyond currently fashionable rhetoric about 'seamless services' and 'total quality' to learn something of how cancer services are encountered by those they ultimately serve: the patients. The result gives much scope for a more sensitive approach to individual care and to service organization.

The authors also have an important theoretical purpose. Here they offer a critical appraisal of the current ideas and thinking about the assessment of quality of life in cancer care. This is an area which has attracted much interest in recent years and where a good deal of effort has gone into the production of measurement scales and instruments of various kinds. Costain Schou and Hewison express major doubts about this work, finding within it an inappropriate emphasis on the functional, the cognitive, the individualistic and the pathological. Such measures, they argue, fail to encompass the essential social context (cultural and structural) in which treatment takes place. Readers must decide to what extent the authors' own methodology can supplant that which they criticize. Certainly it will give encouragement to those involved in quality of life assessment who seek to give greater emphasis to the patient's own priorities and definitions. Perhaps more significantly, the book succeeds as a demonstration of the huge advances which have taken place in qualitative research in recent years, and provides what the authors call a 'nitty gritty' portrayal of the world of cancer treatment, from the patient's perspective.

Experiencing Cancer is the second volume to appear in the Facing Death series. Here it makes two important contributions. First, it reveals how the series will contribute to wider theoretical debates surrounding life-threatening illness and end of life care. This is a growing area of interest in the social and human sciences. Second, it provides a valuable counterpoint to the first volume in the series, *New Themes in Palliative Care* (Clark, Hockley and Ahmedzai 1997). *New Themes* dealt with current ideas and concepts relating to the global development of palliative care, focusing on issues of service development and clinical models. *Experiencing Cancer* provides the voice of the user, suggesting how far we have to go before the theory and practice of high quality cancer care can be brought into line with each other.

David Clark

References

Chief Medical Officers' Expert Advisory Group on Cancer (1995) *A Policy Framework for Commissioning Cancer Services* (the Calman-Hine Report). London: Department of Health.

Clark, D., Hockley, J. and Ahmedzai, A. (1997) *New Themes in Palliative Care*. Buckingham: Open University Press.

Richards, M.A. (1997) Calman-Hine: two years on. *Palliative Medicine*, 11: 433–4.

Acknowledgements

Our deepest gratitude goes to all those who agreed to give their time and their stories for this research at a most difficult period of their lives. Without their willing contributions this work would not have been possible. In the course of this research, several people became dear friends. We would like to dedicate this work to all those who took part, and in particular to the memories of BB and AW.

Introduction

The experience of treatment for cancer is an exhausting, time- and energy-consuming, complex and often confusing process. This book aims to give a detailed expression of this experience, in particular its social nature, as constructed in the interview accounts of a heterogeneous group of newly diagnosed cancer patients. Through these accounts, quality of life in treatment is seen to be largely a function of the quality of care in treatment.

Chapter 1 provides a critical overview of quality of life and psychosocial oncology work. The dominance of a 'functional living' model in quality of life studies, and of a cognitive, individualistic, pathology-oriented focus in psychosocial oncology have led to lack of adequate consideration of the social aspects of the cancer illness experience. Included in the latter are aspects of the health care system and its impact on patients' and families' quality of life, the social conditions subsuming this system and their impact, the impact on the family, treatment experience itself and especially treatment as a social situation, and the need for more contextual research on illness experience and health care settings.

In Chapter 2, this focus on the asocial and individualistic nature of psychosocial oncology is continued with a discussion of the 'antiseptic', asocial view of treatment presented in much of the literature on treatment in psychosocial oncology, with particular reference to studies of diagnosis experience. Many such studies reveal a lack of concern for the social contexts of diagnostic encounters, and how the social situation of diagnosis is constructed through language. Instead, language is viewed non-problematically as a purely referential medium. In the psychosocial literature on diagnostic and treatment experience there is a pervasive location of problems and difficulties in the patient, not in the social situation that effectively and actually *is* 'diagnosis' and 'treatment'.

An alternative view of treatment – as social interaction – is then introduced through the introduction of the empirical material that is a main feature of the book discussion, and developed in subsequent chapters. This material is composed of interview accounts from newly diagnosed patients attending a large regional treatment centre in the north of England. Chapter 2 provides a vivid portrait of the historical and social context of the treatment centre and its work, as depicted in interview excerpts from patients. Also, major themes common to both lay and professional accounts of treatment and of cancer itself are discussed. The importance of these excerpts *as* accounts is highlighted in this chapter, with a focus on how they reflect dominant accounts from the popular media and from within medicine itself, the past experience of patients, and their current experience of the treatment centre. Elements of the social context of the centre are discussed, including the 'ambiguous awareness' context attending many interactions within it, relationships between staff and patients, the organization of the centre, and the types of work involved.

Whereas Chapter 2 introduces the institutional and historical context of treatment for the group of patients whose accounts form the empirical focus of the book, Chapter 3 introduces the general conceptual context of treatment for cancer as a set of calendars to be negotiated and managed by both professionals and patients. The illness calendar (comprised of all appointments, reviews, checks etc.) is the context for all the discrete treatment calendars to which the patient is subjected; treatment calendars are large components of the illness calendar. The early illness calendar, the phase before the start of the treatment calendar (although major surgery forms part of this context for many patients), is dominated by diagnostic processes and prognostic assessments.

The calendar is discussed here as an organizing image for all aspects of the cancer illness experience. The calendar in mainstream Western culture is a linear system of time organization and one that contains markers of general cultural and community context. Calendars also embody goals and represent limitations commonly held within a specific social context. The activity of constructing and 'keeping' calendars is a cultural practice directed at ensuring continuity and predictability in life experience. The experiential and social domains of treatment experience are conceptualized in the book in terms of several types of interrelated calendars: the personal or private, life, illness and treatment calendars. The management of resources in these various calendars by both professionals and patients and the impact of this management on quality of life in treatment are major themes running through the presentation of treatment experience in the book. These resources are broadly defined as those of energy, time, attention, money and space.

The work patients do within the various types of calendars is discussed, alongside a presentation of the often complex, non-linear process of diagnosis, as described by patients in interview accounts. Diagnosis is depicted as a definitional problem for patients, involving much interpretation by individual patients of the 'seriousness' of the illness situation within a context of medical and discursive ambiguity. The pragmatic emphasis in the medical setting is seen to lead potentially to the discounting of issues and concerns that fall outside the immediate medical agenda, but that may be central to quality of life in treatment.

Chapter 4 moves from the context of diagnosis (which frequently involves extensive surgery) to the preparation phases of the radiotherapy and/or chemotherapy treatment calendar(s) that often follow surgery. During this preparation or prescription phase, many patients are recovering from the effects of surgery while they learn about the likely impact of the adjuvant treatment to come. Issues of planning for daily life during the course of treatment, and of prognosis and awareness, are all central concerns at this time. Patients must mobilize local resources for dealing with the rigours of the treatment calendar while coping with losses of function caused by surgery. Identifying and locating the various professionals involved in the treatment calendar(s) in a meaningful context is a major task for patients and family members at this stage of treatment.

Chapter 5 focuses on the experience of post-surgical treatment and the work (by both professionals and patients) of the treatment calendar. Patients' accounts of the different modes of treatment are explored, alongside their struggle to understand the logic of the treatment calendar and any change within it that may occur in the course of treatment. The process of being treated is highlighted, and patients' work in the treatment calendar discussed, including that of interpreting and managing the effects of treatment and attending reviews. The 'costliness' of treatment for patients at this stage, in terms of physical effects, the impact of treatment's substances and processes on the resource of energy, and the rigours of the treatment calendar, are the main conditions influencing quality of life for patients in treatment.

Chapter 6 reviews the key ideas about quality of life of cancer patients in treatment that are discussed in the book, with reference to related literature in three broad areas: health economics and resources rationalization, management in health care, and social support. Aspects of treatment that will have the greatest psychosocial impact will often have more to do with and be more influenced by aspects of the treatment calendar than by either illness or treatment in themselves. Quality of care is seen here chiefly to involve the maximization of time and energy resources for patients in treatment. This main task could be realized through improved management by professionals leading to greater continuity in the experience of treatment; the recognition of 'social support' as an issue inherent in the contexts of treatment (not simply a 'private' issue of personal support 'networks'); the replacement of the individualistic focus of biomedicine and psychosocial oncology with a genuine recognition of treatment as social interaction; and a commitment to studying and improving the social contexts of illness and treatment.

1 Cancer and the quality of life: psycho(social) oncology and the medical model

Introduction

The core of this book consists of a qualitative look at the day-to-day of cancer treatment, focusing on a heterogeneous group of cancer patients attending a large regional treatment centre in northern England. We begin in this chapter with a critical review of two related areas within oncology – the conceptualization and measurement of 'quality of life', and the study of psychosocial aspects of cancer and its treatment. Our critical approach to these two bodies of work on cancer patients is to highlight the lack of attention to the *social* nature of cancer and its treatment, and accordingly to the experience of treatment, quality of care and survivorship issues in much of the psychosocial literature on cancer patients.

The issues raised in the presentation of interview material that follows this chapter are those directly pertaining to the experience of treatment *as* social interaction. Among these are patient and family involvement in treatment (particularly the work they do in the treatment calendar); choice or lack of choice in the treatment situation; information; continuity of care; and the drain on 'personal' resources posed by treatment, especially 'psychosocial' resources of time, energy and attention. The impact of this drain on identity and on the personal calendars of patients is of particular interest. Our dependence on patients' and spouses' accounts of life in treatment is meant to give a vivid impression of the contexts and processes involved in treatment, as well as some of the problems and concerns voiced by patients living the treatment calendar, not all of which may be solvable, but which need acknowledgement.

The focus of these accounts is very much on the 'nitty gritty' detail of daily life for these cancer patients, and it is hoped that the resulting picture of treatment experience will highlight contextual issues that relate to practice. Areas for improvement in the quality of care of patients in treatment that have to do with the health care system itself are highlighted. Relatively small but significant changes in the way in which patients are 'managed' within this system are implicated in our discussion. Several main areas are improving consistency and continuity in the treatment experience through a more coherent treatment calendar management; more 'openness' and better information about the shape (and meaning) of treatment plans; more attention to problems of daily living of persons in treatment; and closer involvement of senior professionals in the management of such problems.

The emergence of the quality of life concept in oncology

Oncology was one of the first areas in medicine to include quality of life on the treatment agenda, because of the low cure rate for most cancers, and the highly toxic nature of many treatments for cancer. Quality of life emerged as a central oncologic topic in the late 1970s and 1980s in part because of an explosion of growth in medical technology aimed at treating cancer and the increasingly complex treatment decisions that have ensued (Maguire and Selby 1989). Technological advancements in medicine led to people with chronic illnesses being kept alive longer, which meant there was a greater, and growing number of chronically ill – a situation that remains today (Gerhardt 1990).

Chronic illness entered the biomedical agenda through the changing character of patient populations in 'acute care' institutions like general hospitals, and through the first qualitative studies of chronic illness in the emerging subdiscipline of medical sociology (Conrad 1990; Gerhardt 1990). The first of these, entitled *Chronic Illness and the Quality of Life* (Strauss and Glaser 1975), argued that much of the work of acute-care institutions was in fact to manage acute phases of chronic illnesses. Ten years later, Strauss *et al.* (1985) described how contemporary medicine, through its power to extend survival, had not only produced new chronic illnesses and phases of illness, but also new kinds of chronically ill people. These people continued to work, have families, and so forth within the now much-changed experience of chronic illness. Thus the 'discovery' in biomedicine of chronic illness at this time set the foundations for the appearance of quality of life as a *biomedical* issue.

Amid the unprecedented technological developments in medicine there were fears about the dehumanizing effects of increasing medicalization on everyday life (Illich 1976) and in the experience of illness (Levanthal *et al.* 1982). The biomedical model (with its emphasis on acute illness) was criticized for its inability to deal with chronicity, and with the experience of illness, and there were calls for a new multidimensional model that could take account of the patient as well as the disease (Engel 1977; Cunningham 1986). Lastly, the rise of the hospice movement in the late 1960s and early 1970s facilitated investigation of the quality of survival of patients with chronic illness. The definition of 'treatment' was expanded to include palliation in the absence of cure, and the illness and symptom management central to life with chronic illness.

The assessment of quality of life in clinical trials of cancer treatments began in the mid-1970s and increased rapidly after 1976 (Selby and Robertson 1986). While survival rates for several cancers have improved as a result of advances in treatment technology, mortality rates have remained largely unaltered for the majority of cancers, and it has become increasingly important to assess the quality as well as the length of survival (Fallowfield 1990). Quality of life assessment is intended to complement the goals of cure and prolongation of life in oncologic treatment (Jones et al. 1987). The central purpose of introducing quality of life endpoints into clinical trials is to add to the traditional ones of general survival, disease-free survival and tumour response (Moinpour et al. 1989). In short, quality of life measurement is a formal attempt at including the patient as well as the disease in the assessment of treatments.

The uses of quality of life information

Despite its acknowledged importance, the impact of quality of life research on clinical practice and treatment decision making is still minimal (Donovan et al. 1989; Traynor 1992). Despite much discussion over the inclusion of quality of life assessment in clinical trials, quality of life has not been a routine trial component, owing initially to a lack of information about the adequacy and relative merits of different measures (Donovan et al. 1989). More recently, it has been pointed out that there is a gap between theory and practice in quality of life assessment in clinical trials, with many of the real-world challenges of assessment inadequately attended to despite the presence of accessible and detailed information about measures and research protocols (Hopwood 1996).

In addition, there is a lack of work on the impact of information about quality of life on accrual of trial results and patient participation in trials as well as in treatment decision making, and there is an array of inconsistent results on whether or not patients are willing to sacrifice survival for quality of life gain from various treatment options (Gotay 1991). The need to synthesize results of clinical trials so as to contribute to clinical practice has been hampered by both the multiplicity of measures and the lack of clear conceptual accounts for many measures, as well as broad variations in assessment practice. Lastly, while there has been increased interest in assessing the quality of care over the past decade (van der Waal *et al.* 1996) and 'strong support' for the view that there should be some relationship between the quality of care and the quality of life (Rosser 1993), aspects of the health care system that directly impact on care and treatment experience are absent from the majority of quality of life studies.

There are many potential uses for quality of life measurement and data. Concern about lack of funding for psychosocial and behavioural cancer research and the defection of many patients from orthodox medicine to 'alternative' or complementary approaches has brought some psychosocial oncologists to press for more attention to quality of life, and to urge clinicians to consider the needs of patients that 'concern their quality of life regardless of treatment's effectiveness' (Burish 1991: 864). In the US, functional status assessments made through quality of life measurement can prevent workplace discrimination against cancer patients. Quality of life surveys may highlight problems that patients take more seriously than physicians, like low back pain. Quality of life assessment in clinical practice could lead to more formal collection and dissemination of information in hospital databases (Deyo 1991).

Quality of life data could be used to help improve clinicians' management of individual patients by helping them to anticipate problems and raise these in discussions with patients; to inform patients of common reactions and aid patients' decision making; and to train staff (Meyerowitz 1993). Routine assessment of patients' quality of life through the disease course would better facilitate the aims of palliative care by allowing more time for intervention (O'Boyle and Waldron 1997). Adult survivors of childhood cancers represent a unique population for whom the long-term impact of treatment on quality of life is a crucial issue. Assessing the quality of survival for long-term survivors of cancer can help target interventions and ultimately inform modifications in treatment (Jenney 1996). Quality of life measurement has emerged as a central aspect of the evaluation of new drugs, both in terms of their effects on patients and cost-benefit analyses, via quality of life-derived instruments like the QALY (Barnett 1991). The uses of quality of life data are wide-ranging and have implications for political and resource allocation issues within the health care arena.

Defining the scope of quality of life in oncology

Definitions of quality of life differ widely (de Haes and van Knippenberg 1985). The World Health Organization's definition of health as physical, mental and social well-being and not merely the absence of disease or infirmity (Nagpal and Sell 1985) dates from 1946 (it was first published in 1958; Bowling 1997), and seems to have informed most attempts at definition of quality of life in the oncologic literature. This definition emphasizes the multidimensional nature of health and well-being and the importance of both positive and negative factors. Two main areas of consensus can be found in the literature on quality of life in oncology: first, that 'quality of life' is a broad term and that conceptual vagueness and the multiplicity of operationalizations of the concept make comparability of studies a problem; and second, that quality of life is a multidimensional concept, inclusive of the psychological and social as well as of the physical (Jenkins *et al.* 1990; Aaronson *et al.* 1991; Bloom 1991; Hopwood 1992).

In the traditional biomedical model that continues to dominate medical practice, physicians and caregivers set goals for patients and then assess progress (Joyce 1988). 'Quality of life' assessment is an attempt at expanding this clinical view to include the patient's assessment of treatment's impact. This attempt at including the patient's perspective is in conflict with the need to have clear and concise measures so as not to interrupt the 'flow' of the time-pressed clinic, and to reduce patient burden. Emphasis on the latter concerns has led to a retention of the biomedical focus on pathology, on symptoms and functioning, and on aspects of treatment's impact most relevant to the clinical trial, such as symptom control, maintenance of mobility, physical independence and psychological distress.

An increasing gap has emerged between the sophistication of statistical analysis aimed at quality of life questionnaire data and the lack of *conceptual* sophistication reflected in the operationalization of the factors or areas of concern contributing to quality of life (MacDowell and Newell 1987; Bowling 1997). Connected with this problem is that of overly complex reporting in many quality of life studies, including unnecessary sophistication in the analysis of quality of life data, coupled with poor study design (Montazeri *et al.* 1996). Generally, quality of life is operationalized as functional status across various domains of functioning (Aaronson *et al.* 1988; Holland 1992b). It can be argued that quality of life assessment in oncology retains its essentially biomedical focus through an implicit dependence on a 'functional living' perspective (Schipper *et al.* 1984 and Schipper 1990 give an explicit description of this model). This dominant conceptualization of quality of life is taken from early performance status measures and independent activities of daily living scales (MacDowell and Newell 1987). 'Health-related' quality of life may be extended to include other dimensions of life, such as financial status (Deyo 1991), but non-function-specific concerns get little mention in the quality of life literature. Under the rubric of functional living are concerns about physical and psychological morbidity, and the capacity of the patient for active and independent functioning.

In focusing almost exclusively on physical, psychological and active role *functioning*, quality of life researchers have focused on pathology, and essentially restricted the study of psychosocial aspects of cancer to attempts at detecting psychopathology and measuring levels of distress among patients.

It has been pointed out however that the quality of *life* and the quality of function are not necessarily the same thing (Chaturvedi 1991). What is neglected within this paradigm is any notion of the *meaning* of the experience of cancer and treatment for the individual patient. One recent approach that addresses this limitation by employing an individual perspective to the definition and assessment of quality of life is the SEIQoL, or the Schedule for the Evaluation of Individual Quality of Life (O'Boyle 1994). The schedule is based on judgement analysis and allows the individual respondent to weight the relative importance of self-identified areas of experience and to assess how they are doing in relation to each one. In this way the unique perspective of the individual forms the basis of every aspect of the assessment, which provides readily interpretable information for use in the clinical management of the patient.

Beyond the presence or absence of function, 'meaning' may include issues of *understanding* and acknowledgement from professionals (not mere levels of information 'received' by patients), ideas about supportive and non-supportive contact with professionals and others, the nature of choice in treatment, and changing definitions of 'ordinary' experience as the treatment trajectory continues, or is brought to an end. There have been calls for a movement beyond the 'distress' focus in psychosocial oncology, and toward the exploration of meaning in the experience of illness and treatment (Morse and Johnson 1991; Fife 1994 and 1995; Mathiesen and Stam 1995; Bowling 1997). More recently, there has been explicit acknowledgement of the importance of phenomenological and spiritual determinants of quality of life in the appearance of several measures that address these issues, such as the McGill Quality of Life Questionnaire, and the Life Evaluation Questionnaire (cited in O'Boyle and Waldron 1997). One area in which such dimensions assume prime importance is that of palliative care (although there has been a lack of empirical work on quality of life in palliative care; O'Boyle and Waldron 1997). However, others have argued that 'pragmatism' should be the central determinant of quality of life in oncology (Patrick and Erickson 1988; Faden and LePlege 1992), and there is much tension between the goal of placing the patient's experience at the centre of quality of life assessment, and that of streamlining such assessment to fit easily within the practical limitations of the clinic or the clinical trial.

Beyond the care of the individual patient however (and it is here that quality of life assessment has had the least impact) there is an increasing and sometimes indiscriminate use of quality of life measures for ever-broadening purposes, such as the distribution of health service resources, and the audit of clinical practice (Cox *et al.* 1992), making the issues of choice and suitability of measures for different settings and uses more important. Currently, a 'core' quality of life measure is favoured, supplemented by disease-specific modules, and since the 1980s, the Study Group on Quality of Life within the European Organization for Research and Treatment of Cancer (EORTC) has been developing a self-assessment core questionnaire that is multi-dimensional, cancer-specific and cross-culturally validated (Sigurdardottir *et al.* 1996). However, 'narrowing' of either the quality of life construct or the number of measures used to assess it does not in itself resolve dilemmas over the *meaning* of 'quality of life' (Faden and LePlege 1992).

Psychosocial oncology and quality of life

Since the late 1970s and early 1980s there has been a growing awareness of the role of psychological factors in the onset, development, treatment and handling of cancer (Watson and Morris 1985; Beckmann 1989; Somerfield and Curbow 1992). Psychosocial oncology has been an emerging sub-discipline in oncology for the past 15 years (Holland 1992a; Somerfield and Curbow 1992). There has been pressure from within psychosocial oncology for the 'scientific' measurement of psychosocial factors and quality of life through questionnaires (Dreher 1987) and for such measurement to become a standard part of clinical trials research and clinical practice.

Early research in the 1950s to early 1970s was largely anecdotal and psychoanalytic in perspective (Hopwood and Maguire 1988; Somerfield and Curbow 1992). Questionnaire studies in the 1970s and 1980s focused on high levels of psychological or psychiatric morbidity (anxiety and depression) in cancer patients (Greer and Morris 1975; Morris *et al.* 1977; Derogatis *et al.* 1983). The literature on the prevalence of depression and anxiety in cancer patients is conflicting, with studies reporting anywhere from 5 to 50 per cent or more of cancer patients as identifiable cases. Potential reasons for the underdiagnosis of depression in cancer patients are the use of restrictive definitions of the term, or the confounding of organic indicators with the effects of the disease itself (Spiegel 1997). However, it has been suggested that psychological morbidity in cancer patients has been overestimated and that there has been an overemphasis on the negative experience of quality of life (Meyerowitz 1993; Bowling 1997). Rates of depression and depressive states for cancer in-patients are comparable to those reported for patients with other diagnoses with a similar level of illness (Spiegel 1997). Many studies deal only with patients who have already been diagnosed as cases of psychiatric morbidity, and clinical dependence on such work encourages a one-dimensional view of cancer patients and the experience of cancer and its treatment. Along with the emphasis on functioning in quality of life, the casting of the personal experience of illness in terms of 'psychosocial morbidity' medicalizes and pathologizes this experience.

Survivorship appears to have been a neglected area in psychosocial oncology and quality of life research, although it is a major topic in the supportive care literature, particularly in the US. Auchincloss (1995), for example, found few descriptive studies relevant to the 'psychological terrain' of the long-term gynaecologic cancer survivor. Jenney (1996), speaking about long-term survivors of childhood cancers, points out that as survival rates improve for some cancers, doctors and patients will need to be given reliable information about the impact of treatments on quality of life in the long term, as well as about the relative success of different treatments. The lack of survivorship studies can be linked to the relatively poor rates of survival still associated with many cancers, but psychosocial and quality of life concerns following treatment, however long or short any post-treatment period may be, remain central concerns affecting the daily lives of patients and families. There appears to be something of a gap between the psychosocial oncology literature and the supportive and palliative care literature, in that they appear to be distinct areas of concern to two distinct groups of professionals. There has been a drive toward professionalization in psychosocial oncology, to establish it as a subdiscipline of oncology. This has perhaps kept those involved expressly within it, working alongside oncologists at the 'front lines' of treatment, from adequate cooperation with those counsellors, social workers, special care nurses and patient advocates working within supportive care. For these latter professionals, issues of survivorship, advanced disease and quality of care are central concerns, though they are given little voice in the psychosocial literature *per se*. There has been interest in supportive care interventions for cancer patients since the 1970s, though psychosocial oncologists have been less obviously concerned with these than with charting distress in cancer patients and exploring links between stress and personality factors and prognosis. Currently, however, there is greater interest in the role of such interventions (the four main types being behavioural therapy, educational therapy, psychotherapy, and support groups; Fallowfield 1995) for patients and their families in improving quality of life, coping, compliance, and even survival in cancer patients (Bloch and Kissane 1995; Fallowfield 1995; Spiegel 1997). Perhaps these recent calls to make supportive therapy a routine part of cancer treatment plans will mean that issues related to supportive care will begin to enjoy more attention from psychosocial oncologists.

Two main categories of concerns in psychosocial oncology are clinical studies of psychosocial effects of cancer and its treatment, including clinical trials of psychosocial therapies, and the role of stress and personality in the etiology and progression of the disease (Greer 1987). Included here are studies of the connection between psychological and biological mechanisms in the development of cancer (Holland 1992a). Studies of the contexts of the experience of treatment are scarce. The 'social' aspect of psychosocial oncology refers mostly to the emotional responses of patients and others close to the disease and the effect of these responses on relationships (Holland 1992a), though the impact on the family is frequently not included

(Moynihan 1991; Davis-Ali *et al.* 1993). Also included under this rubric is the quantity and quality of 'social support' available to the patient (Aaronson *et al.* 1988), and the patient's capacity for 'role functioning' (Bloom 1991). These concerns underscore the 'functional status' focus within psychosocial oncology. Psychosocial oncology is heavily dominated by a focus on psycho-pathology (Mathiesen and Stam 1995) and has even been called 'psychiatric oncology' (Greer 1987).

Psychological aspects in quality of life measures and studies of psycho-social dimensions of treatment are most often defined in relation to the functional living perspective described earlier. In this perspective, the degree of 'distress' felt by the patient is assessed, both as an outcome of treatment, and as a prognostic indicator (linking 'coping styles', loosely the ability to deal with 'distress' and stress, to prognosis for example) (Silberfarb *et al.* 1980; Fobair and Mages 1981; Zigmond and Snaith 1983; Beckmann 1989). Psychosocial oncology also espouses an asocial, philosophical individual-ism that arises out of its connection with biomedicine.

This emphasis on individualism originates in the biomedical model of disease and treatment which shapes medical practice. In the biomedical model, disease processes are considered identifiable as 'entities' through a reductionist process of isolating linear cause and effect relationships in specific diseased organs. Emphasis is placed on the affected part and the nature of the disease involvement in the body, so that interventions can be targeted. In this perspective in psychosocial studies, the bounded entity of the individual, separated from social context, is the focus of study, with the eventual 'summing together' of individuals' behaviour, reactions, beliefs, etc. comprising the results of studies. Ironically, this individualistic focus has not translated into practical use in the treatment and medical manage-ment of individual *patients*, perhaps because in such research it is the (re-constructed) context of the *summary* of individuals that is of interest (the greater the number of individuals, the more valid and reliable the results). Also, this individualistic focus locates the source of 'experience', reactions, problems, coping etc. *inside* the individual patient (rather than outside, in the social world of the treatment institution, for example). Thus, the study of personality 'types' and coping styles in the onset and/or progression of cancer; the relationship between psychological responses, disease progres-sion, prognosis, and reaction to treatment; and patients' self-esteem, body image and sexuality are several common topics of study, whereas studies of health care contexts are virtually nonexistent. Under this rubric, for example, improving doctor–patient relationships in order to influence adjustment positively is cast in terms of the need to reduce patient anxiety, as well as bolster patient optimism by being aware of 'information that would make a patient unduly pessimistic [,] increase thought intrusion and reduce life satisfaction' (Spiegel 1997; S1–38). There is an implicit suggestion here that information control is seen as a legitimate means of protecting optimism in patients. As long as the problem and its solution are seen to reside forever *in* the patient, such dangerous justifications will continue to be an underlying message of psychosocial oncology.

'Coping' in psychosocial oncology

Allied with the study of psychological distress and morbidity in psychosocial oncology is the study of 'coping'. Coping is among the most widely studied psychosocial factors in research on cancer patients (Somerfield and Curbow 1992). There has recently been a shift away from static approaches to 'coping' (as an unconscious response to inner conflict) to conceptualizations that focus on coping as an active and conscious response to situational stressors (Somerfield and Curbow 1992), and 'role functioning' as well as to cognitive and affective *state* (Bloom *et al.* 1992). The current view is that it is not 'stress' itself, but individuals' specific behavioural and biological responses to stress that contribute to the development and the progress of cancer (Cull 1990).

Self-report questionnaires like the Hospital Anxiety and Depression Scale (HADS) and the Rotterdam Symptom Checklist (RSCL) are used increasingly to assess the quality of life of patients, with a focus on psychological functioning and distress. Given the difficulty of placing results in context, and of interpreting them for the individual patient, caution has been urged in the interpretation of questionnaire results (Breetvelt and van Dam 1991; Cox *et al.* 1992). The HADS and the RSCL, for example, have been found to be limited in their capacity to distinguish true cases (as defined in a psychiatric interview) from other respondents with high 'distress' scores (Hopwood *et al.* 1991a). Use of such measures to screen for psychiatric disorders has been defended on pragmatic grounds (Hopwood *et al.* 1991b), and with a view to targeting interventions, like cognitive–behavioural therapy, to help patients overcome their distress (Greer *et al.* 1992).

Psychosocial oncology and quality of life studies share similar methodological problems. The most striking aspect of psychosocial research in oncology is the apparent inconsistency of findings between studies (Temoshok and Heller 1984; Beckmann 1989; Liang *et al.* 1990). This appears bound up in the heterogeneity of studies in relation to definitions of outcome, different study designs, and different measures and forms of measure, all hindering comparability (Temoshok and Heller 1984). Two general criticisms that can be made are that research conclusions are heavily reliant on correlational evidence, and that this evidence is weak. Also, the majority of studies are on women with breast cancer, and caution has been urged in generalization of results from one cancer population to another (Davis-Ali *et al.* 1993).

Biomedical individualism and 'health behaviour'

A major criticism of psychosocial oncology and quality of life research is that, in retaining an essentially biomedical, individualistic perspective, and focusing on 'health behaviour' and behavioural change, such work excludes important features of the experience of illness that involve the social, institutional and political contexts of cancer patients and their families. Moynihan (1987: 487) points out that the 'massive upsurge' of interest in psychosocial research in the 1980s was 'concomitant with a philosophy of individualism which, in turn, is embraced by the neoconservative ideology' of the times, and is still in evidence in the late 1990s.

Psychosocial oncology shares with the cancer research establishment (as represented by the major cancer research organizations in both the US and Britain) primary concerns of 'detection, prevention and compliance' (Holland 1992a). Following this perspective, Holland (1992a: 11) articulates the stance of psycho-oncology towards prevention:

> Ability to change attitudes and behaviour constitutes the chief way to control development of neoplasms which are dependent upon exposure to carcinogens. Social scientists provide the resource to examine how to change behaviours related to sun exposure, smoking and occupational exposures.

Importantly, this perspective encourages the minimization of aspects of illness experience that do not originate from *within* the person. Other aspects of the illness experience besides personal behaviour, like the health care system (however this system is constituted in different countries) and structural factors affecting the quality of care and access to resources, are frequently omitted. Those emanating from the larger sociocultural context that subsumes both patient and health care system are also largely unattended to, receiving at best a 'cursory nod' (Moynihan 1987).

Mathiesen and Stam (1995) point out that the individualism of psychosocial oncology is supported in large part by dependence on a model of cognitive adaptation characterized by the maintenance of sharp distinctions between self and others as a requirement of psychological health, with high internal control the ideal. Such a view, the authors observe, casts cancer as 'a personal problem to be solved, mainly through the adoption of appropriate coping strategies' (1995: 286). With its heavily cognitive bias, the 'social' aspect of psychosocial oncology is mainly located in the individual responses of patients.

In interpreting the individualism of psychosocial oncology, it is important to note that the growth of this 'subspecialty' has been largely contingent on its remaining close to the biomedical world (characterized by a 'clinical mentality' of individualism; Friedson 1970) of the oncology establishment.[1] In order to achieve a power base, workers in the field have concentrated on demonstrating their right to a central (rather than fringe) place in oncology, by addressing biomedical concerns, and convincing clinicians that the skills of psycho-oncology (essentially, psychometrics and counselling/therapy approaches) are both unique and useful. This has meant a focus on the 'hardness' and thus legitimacy of questionnaire research, a pragmatic emphasis on traditional clinical endpoints, and the tantalizing prospect of new ways to demonstrate treatment effectiveness.

Criticisms of the individualistic, 'behavioural' focus in psychosocial oncology and health psychology have been made. In 1978, Levine and Kozloff concluded it was time to move beyond the Parsonian 'sick role' model of health and illness, to studies of the social behaviour of ill people and how the 'larger political and economic order' was related to personal behaviour. More recently, Mechanic (1992) has observed that in the US, the concept of health as a community responsibility has been all but 'demolished', in favour of cost-efficiency concerns and a market philosophy, with a corresponding lack of attention paid to structural and political constraints on 'health behaviour'. He calls for a reconceptualization of the problems facing disabled people and their families, from being 'personal health problems' to being linked to issues of discrimination and blocked opportunities.

Also, the organization of medical *practice* may be as important in the success of the patient–physican interaction as the personal characteristics of either participant. Clinical issues, because they deal with the management of expertise and knowledge, are *power* issues; they are thus political issues as well, and are central to such concerns as 'patient satisfaction', that tend to hinge on the provision and communication of information in the clinical encounter (Carr-Hill 1992). Medical sociologists in Britain have commented on how the 'consumer rights' individualism stressed in the 1989 White Paper did not result in greater choice for patients although it stressed greater personal responsibility for health (Elston 1991; Mohan 1991).

The challenge to an 'asocial' psychosocial oncology

In the 1980s and 1990s, there has been intellectual criticism of biomedicine as well as an increasing tendency in the general population to turn to complementary medicine for help (Sharma 1990; Stainton-Rogers 1991). The inclusion also of 'holistic' health practices among some orthodox practitioners and the increasing public interest in 'alternative therapies' for cancer and other chronic illnesses (Pietroni 1990) point to continuing challenges to orthodox medicine. In addition to growing critical discourse about biomedicine, there has been a corresponding growth of 'self-help' movements for the chronically ill and disabled (Mechanic 1992; Ritchie

1992). Such groups are gradually becoming more involved in the political issues of chronic illness and disability.

If patients' actions challenge or obstruct the biomedical goals of disease management, or the goals of the organization within which this work occurs, they are prone to interpretation in terms of an 'illness as deviance' focus (Gerson 1976). It can be argued that this conceptualization of illness as deviance (arising from Parsons's 'sick role' model and the 'sickness behaviour' perspective) is reconstituted in psychosocial oncology primarily as the failure to 'cope' well. In contrast, other authors have underscored the necessity of linking the 'local worlds' of individuals to larger social processes and organizational contexts. For example, Anderson et al. (1991: 108), in a study comparing Chinese and Anglo-Canadian women's perspectives on chronic illness, state that individual differences in 'reconstructing life' and managing illness have to be viewed not only as ethnic differences, but also in terms of class differences, and those related to 'how social processes organize the experience of illness'. They note that

> Dominant ideologies are interwoven into, and are reproduced in on-going social interactions; they are used to assess how well one is doing. For example, tacit knowledge about the value of 'inner strength' and 'taking responsibility for self', provide the background for interactions in the patient–practitioner encounter.
>
> (Anderson et al. 1991: 111)

These ideological frameworks 'permeate the health care system'.

Similarly, Clark et al. (1991: 818) call for an analysis of clinical decision making in its social contexts (although part of their focus is on the personal and social 'characteristics' of patients) not to 'control or eliminate social factors that might "interrupt" technically efficient standardized care' but to 'underscore the irremediably social, and human nature of medical care'. In a recent study of verbal interaction on a leukaemia ward, for example, the ward is described primarily as a social setting prone to 'legitimacy problems' (based mainly on the fact that the treatment work of the ward causes most of the 'illness' experience of the patients). Work done in spoken interaction needs to be explicitly acknowledged by professionals and not seen merely as the relaying of *fact*, or 'information'. Simiroff and Fetting (1991) also highlight the social nature of health care and the political implications of 'information' in the doctor–patient relationship, noting in their study that patients with more specific information from physicians may choose to make decisions that run counter to those of professionals. These studies move beyond the properties of patients as individuals to address explicitly the social and political issues involved in the health care setting.

Focusing on the meaning of the illness experience (in both practical and existential terms) is something that has been undertaken in the self-help

literature, but largely ignored in the stress and coping psychosocial literature (Fife 1994 and 1995). Fife (1995: 1022) defines 'meaning' in chronic
illness as 'the individual's understanding of the implications an illness has
for his/her identity and for the future . . . individuals' perceptions of their
ability to accomplish future goals, to maintain the viability of interpersonal
relationships, and to sustain a sense of personal vitality, competence and
power'. We would add that the construction of meaning is not merely
'cognitive' and a matter of 'individuals' perceptions', but a *social* process
achieved by people in relationship within specific 'local worlds' (Kleinman
1992).

Bury, in a review of sociological research on chronic illness, has noted
that the issue of *treatment* and its place in the experience of chronic illness
'has only recently begun to receive the attention it deserves' (Bury 1991:
457). Despite the enthusiasm of psychosocial oncologists for quality of life
measurement, little attention has been paid to the quality of *survival* and
the restoration of functional health following invasive treatment (Olweny
et al. 1993). Failure to pay attention to treatment and recovery experience
can result in unidentified needs both within the treatment context and outside it (MacDonald 1988; Deeny and McCrea 1991; Corney *et al.* 1992),
often resulting in years of suffering after treatment has been completed.
Knowledge of patients' experience of treatment can be used to improve
this experience and to guide health care more effectively. The contexts of
health care are integral to patients' psychosocial experience of treatment,
and psychosocial well-being can be seen to arise from and within the various
relationships between patients and professionals, and through continuity
of care (Guex 1994). A much-neglected but perhaps most important topic,
the impact of the health care system *itself* on patients' 'quality of life' and
treatment experience, must be included in assessments of treatments' impact
(Hietanen 1996).

In addition, the *work* done by patients in treatment has 'only just begun
to be considered in any depth' (Bury 1991: 459). More attention should be
paid to patients' contributions to assessing the quality of care and influencing changes in clinical practice (van der Waal *et al.* 1996). Treatment is
not a passive experience for cancer patients, whose management of its processes and effects plays a large part in its success. Corbin and Strauss (1988:
67) call for a move beyond strictly psychological or psychiatric concepts
such as stress and coping in understanding the problems of patients and
families living with chronic illness. Rather, 'the practitioner requires a set
of concepts allied with observer–interviewer sensitivity that will sensitize
him or her to the combined psychological and social aspects of the chronic
illness experience'. Research on cancer patients in treatment needs to focus
on the basic structures and processes of cancer health care environments
to further understanding of social support and environment (Kobasa *et al.*
1991). 'Treatment' can be defined in terms of these 'basic structures and

processes', although the biomedical view of treatment, implicit in the psychosocial oncology literature, seems to have been one of disconnection from the contexts and work of health care environments.

Methodology is an important issue within that of developing accounts of illness that deal with the socio-cultural levels of the 'illness experience'. The focus in quality of life and psychosocial oncology research has been almost exclusively on questionnaire development and administration. The emphasis on measurement has obscured contextual and definitional issues, and this narrowness has in turn created problems (ironically) for both measurement and the implementation of changes in clinical practice. Also, the acknowledged concern in psychosocial oncology with counselling and other therapeutic approaches is not served by its failure to deal adequately with illness and treatment contexts. Research methodologies that emphasize exploration of context can contribute much to a non-prescriptive counselling approach, as well as shed light on more 'delimited' problems within the arena of counselling.

Much of the work on health care contexts cited here employs methodological approaches that allow for an exploration of context through which the social nature of medical practice is able to appear. Such work focuses on the arena in which institutional and organizational issues meet those of personal meaning and the 'private' experience of illness. The discussion provided in the chapters of this book is intended to be a small contribution to this work. In placing the *contexts* of treatment experience in focus, viewed through the accounts of patients and their families, we have tried to link the personal and the institutional dimensions of treatment experience.

Summary

Quality of life in cancer is still conceptualized largely in terms of a functional living framework in which conventional biomedical concerns have priority. This framework excludes much that is important to the patient and fails to take account of the social and personal contexts of the cancer illness and treatment experiences. Despite the increasing use of quality of life assessment in oncology, there are many methodological and conceptual problems, and little evidence that quality of life information has had much impact on the care of the individual patient. Moving beyond the inherent individualism and 'distress' focus in psychosocial oncology is required in order to include those aspects of quality of life that address the social nature of treatment. Patients' experiences of treatment, of the health care system itself, and of life with cancer following treatment are all aspects of the social experience of illness that require much more attention than they have hitherto received in the psychosocial oncology literature.

Chapter 2 provides a critique of how 'treatment' has been conceptualized in the psychosocial oncology literature, and presents an alternative view of treatment as social interaction. This chapter also introduces the treatment setting and patients involved in the study of treatment experience that is the focus of this book.

Note

1 By 'establishment' we mean both 'oncology', the study of cancer and the study and practice of its treatment, and the funding bodies that carry out cancer research. In Britain, only 12 per cent of cancer research comes from the government. The two largest charities are the Imperial Cancer Research Fund (ICRF) and the Cancer Research Campaign (CRC), which command £50m and £45m per year respectively for cancer research, most of which comes from donations by the public ('Is glamour the best way to treat breast cancer?', *Daily Telegraph*, 3 March 1992).

2 Treatment as social interaction

This chapter will present two views of cancer treatment, one from the psychosocial literature on diagnosis experiences of patients, and a quite different view from our study of treatment experience which is the focus of this book. The interview material in the book was derived from a study of cancer patients' experiences in treatment at a large regional treatment centre and teaching facility in the north of England. A brief description of the study background will be provided here (see the Appendix for a description of the study methodology), followed by a critical discussion of how treatment has been portrayed in the psychosocial literature. After a description of the treatment centre featured in our study, the rest of the chapter will explore the social context of the centre through excerpts from interviews with patients in treatment there. The excerpts and discussion are intended to provide initial context for the view of treatment as social interaction developed in this book, as well as to establish the local context of treatment for this particular group of cancer patients. The material in this chapter will set the scene for the more detailed exploration of treatment as a social process that follows in Chapters 3–5.

The material presented in this book comes from a qualitative study of treatment experiences of a heterogeneous group of 44 cancer patients undergoing radiotherapy and/or chemotherapy at City A regional treatment centre, most for a first diagnosis of cancer. Reference will be made as well to a district hospital at City B, roughly 45 minutes' driving distance from City A, where several patients attended for chemotherapy.[1] Interviews of between one and a half and three and a half hours' length were conducted with patients and their spouses post-diagnosis and before radiotherapy treatment started and several weeks after the treatment schedule was completed, in patients' homes. All interviews were audiotaped and transcribed in full, and analysed using procedures of grounded theory described in Glaser and Strauss (1967) and Strauss and Corbin (1990).[2]

Treatment as an 'antiseptic' process: the case of diagnosis studies

Psychosocial studies of treatment are most usually studies of 'quality of life', in which treatment is predominantly depicted as an anonymous, antiseptic, asocial process taking place independently of individual agents. Treatment processes are assumed to be neutral, except as regards the therapeutic and 'side' effects directly caused by the substances used to treat. These studies share three main features. The first is a (usually implicit) dependence on a functional living perspective such that a high level of physical and psychological functioning equates to high quality of life, which means that variation in patient responses to treatment is likely to be conceptualized in terms of *dys*function or pathology. Second, a definition of psychosocial dysfunction as for the most part arising from patients' own personalities (or poor coping strategies) is common. And third, the assumption is made that descriptions and interview responses from patients can be taken uncritically as evidence for cognitive–behavioural mechanisms and processes through which the patient's 'personality type', 'coping style' or 'reactions' can be accessed. What these studies routinely ignore or underexamine is the *social* nature of the treatment (and indeed, the research) situation, a significant aspect of which is the role of language in the social construction of treatment (and of research accounts of treatment experience).

Studies in the psychosocial oncology literature of patients' reactions to diagnosis offer examples of biomedical constructions of 'treatment'. In these studies, the diagnosis is 'administered' to the patient, and the patient's reactions to this event are extracted from interview and/or questionnaire responses. The biomedical view of the person informs these studies; in this view, illness and disease is located in the person, who is 'bounded by the body', 'wholly separate from the social environment and . . . composed of modules which can be analysed and manipulated in relative isolation' (Spicer and Chamberlain 1996: 166). Admi (1996) summarizes dominant theoretical views of chronic conditions as having been shaped by psychoanalytic thought (the search for psychopathology central to this view), or biomedical perspectives (with pathology and function concerns central). She describes the 'ordinary lifestyle framework' (in which chronic conditions are viewed as background context, not the focus of identity) as an alternative way of viewing chronic illness.

The biomedical model is translated in psychosocial oncology into a psychiatric model of the cancer patient, in studies using psychiatric indices to classify patients according to their emotional reactions to cancer (Mathiesen and Stam 1995). These classifications often result in a high incidence of diagnoses of depression and anxiety, although when non-psychiatric criteria are used, the incidence of such problems falls dramatically (Weisman *et al.* 1980; Wellisch *et al.* 1983; Cassileth *et al.* 1986; cited in Mathiesen and Stam 1995). Other studies suggest that the incidence of anxiety and depression may be quite low even when psychiatric criteria are applied. Two recent examples are a study assessing anxiety experienced by cancer survivors at follow-up appointments one to three years following diagnosis (Nordin *et al.* 1996) which found that less than 20 per cent experienced measurable distress (as assessed by the Hospital Anxiety and Depression scale – HADS), and a study of psychological adjustment to cancer which found that the majority of patients 'coped well' (Rodrigue *et al.* 1994). It is acknowledged that patients' responses to hearing a diagnosis of cancer are various and often seem unpredictable: some people respond with a positive dynamism while others retreat into shock or experience extreme distress, thus exhibiting 'psychosocial morbidity'. Though cancer patients with clinical levels of anxiety and depression are a minority, this is often cast as a problem of detection resulting from physicians' poor interviewing skills (Davenport *et al.* 1987; Ford *et al.* 1996). The aim of the bulk of these studies into diagnosis and treatment experience of cancer patients is to diagnose such 'distress' or 'morbidity' and to target the patient for drug or counselling therapies that are effectively treatments for psychopathology (Mathiesen and Stam 1995).

Patients' responses to diagnosis (seen as equivalent to their responses to questionnaire or interview questions about this experience) are routinely decontextualized in these studies. In one of the first of such studies, exhaustive medical background was provided, demographic data and psychological assessment via a battery of tests was alluded to, and a six-section interview described which approached the task of delineating context (details about beliefs, relationships, understanding information, and so forth), although the manner in which the diagnosis had been delivered was not addressed (Morris *et al.* 1985). Although the effort here had been made to collect detailed data, the interviews were then analysed in such a way as to discount much of this detail. All statements describing emotional and mental 'responses' to diagnosis were extracted, and these were further analysed to reveal cognitive and behavioural responses. Language is seen in most studies of psychosocial experience as a neutral, referential medium that points to phenomena, rather than as the only actual object for analysis itself. In a recent study on doctor–patient interaction during 'bad news consultations' using audiotapes (Ford *et al.* 1996), the reader is assured that 'patients were well-informed about their diagnosis, prognosis and treatment options', but no examples of actual excerpts from the tapes regarding these topics are provided (the study focuses on consultants' failure to elicit psychosocial information through an overly 'closed' and dominating interview style). Rather, 'the diagnosis' ('the bad news') is taken as a given, universally understood entity (although admittedly aspects of the *manner* of physician interaction and of the consultation situation are discussed in this study). The data as *language* are invisible, represented instead by statistical reduction.

In most studies of diagnosis there is a lack of attention to – and often a complete failure to address – the processes comprising the physician's construction of a diagnosis. Even general distinctions, like whether the diagnostic process was fraught with ambiguity and information gaps, complex procedures and conflicting test results, or whether it was smooth, speedy and reached a conclusive result with little ambiguity, are left unacknowledged. 'Diagnosis' for cancer often involves invasive procedures and repeated tests, as well as actual treatment processes (the line between reaching a diagnosis and beginning treatment is often difficult to draw). Questions are often not asked about how the diagnostic information was communicated, the wording used, the content of what was said, the duration of the consultation, and the professional involved. In the early part of the study reported in this book, three of the twenty respondents interviewed at that time described receiving statements of diagnosis from junior registrars, three received them from GPs, and four heard them 'unofficially' from nurses. Also, six of the twenty patients asserted that they had not been expressly told they had cancer. Diagnosis is often discussed as if it were a context-independent entity, rather than the result of interacting context-specific processes comprised of the (inter)actions of individual actors.

Responses to diagnosis and treatment experience are often described as properties of the patient, rather than as responses to the nature of the diagnostic information, or to the diagnostic situation. 'Avoidance (denial)', a 'coping style' featured in one study of diagnosis (Greer *et al.* 1989), refers to 'the minimization of the seriousness' of diagnosis and the denial of anxiety about it. Yet treatment professionals frequently use ways of telling about diagnosis and treatment that minimize the seriousness (implications for prognosis and lasting impairment) of cancer and its treatment. In the study of diagnosis and early treatment experience of cancer patients described in this book, the authors found minimization to be a pervasive communication style for the four consultants involved. They frequently described extensive radiotherapy courses of four to six weeks as 'just a precaution' against the surgeon's 'having missed one or two cells' of the cancer. The word 'cancer' was reported by respondents (all of whom expressed the knowledge that they had cancer) to have been left out roughly half of the time. Several patients were told they had a 'tumour' or 'growth' instead. For example, one elderly patient with extensive cancer of the anal margin was simply told her illness 'would not require a major operation' and was treatable with radiotherapy alone (in fact, she was inoperable and eligible only for palliative radiotherapy to shrink the mass). Another woman was told about her impending mastectomy by her surgeon observing, 'Well, you won't be able to topless sunbathe any more.'

Minimization seemed to be a built-in feature of the treatment situation, from diagnosis onwards. It included the use of 'benign' or ambiguous wording ('growth' instead of 'cancer'), humour and delaying the diagnosis. (In one extreme case of the latter, a patient reported being told only about post-operative treatment options by her surgeon, who refused to state the diagnosis conclusively. He eventually told her she had breast cancer just before she was anaesthetized for a lumpectomy.) There was also a subtle, pervasive 'cheerfulness' which, in addition to the brevity of the consultations, seemed to forestall the expression of emotion or the asking of questions on the part of the patients involved. Other minimizing practices used by diagnostic professionals were the use of junior staff and students to deliver the 'bad news' and the failure to mention the possibility of further post-operative treatment. It appears that minimization is a dominant feature of the diagnostic/treatment context. Proposing to deal primarily with the cognitive–behavioural responses of the patient instead of the context of diagnosis is one way of excluding social context as a topic of analysis.

In locating the source of all difficulty or debate in the patient (the patient's 'responses' to treatment or to a statement of diagnosis) the focus is taken away from aspects of the health care setting, or the actions of specific professionals within it. For example, within this 'behaviour' focus, problems with informed consent in clinical trials can be rearticulated as 'doctors' failures to recognize patients' misconceptions' (Fallowfield 1988). Such formulations encourage a Parsonian focus on the so-called 'competence gap' between doctors and patients (Turner 1995), such that the issue appears to be the improvement of communication skills of doctors, and not the political and ethical issues posed by clinical trials. In professing to look at the 'subjective responses' of patients to treatment and illness (ostensibly an attempt at including the patient as well as the disease in quality of life work) such work can subtly bypass social and political issues of health care in favour of decontextualized arenas of 'interaction'. These are then dealt with more or less exclusively in terms of 'information-processing' or 'coping' abilities, or other idiosyncrasies and deviance of the patient. For example, a study of 'patient satisfaction' with interaction with hospital physicians compared 'patient-rated satisfaction' with an observer-rated checklist of 'physician behaviors' exhibited during ward rounds. The study found that physician behaviours differed widely and yet patient-assessed satisfaction was high. The authors concluded that 'patient satisfaction is more a function of patient perceptions and patient age than of specific physician behaviors' (Blanchard et al. 1990). This increased attention to the 'subjectivity' of the patient in psychosocial oncology and quality of life work can be used to obscure aspects of patients' illness and treatment experience that call the biomedical agenda into question.

Treatment experience at City A regional centre: institutional context

City A treatment centre, located in a large city in the north of England, was a regional radiotherapy centre serving a wide catchment area, also providing chemotherapy and in-patient care for cancer patients undergoing treatment (this description of the centre appears in Costain Schou 1993).[3] Several thousand patients each year were treated on an outpatient basis, with a smaller number treated as in-patients. Most of the patients in this study were receiving radiotherapy as outpatients. Patients were referred to the centre from district or general hospitals, or via specialist clinics held in several regional hospitals by the centre's own consultants. The centre was a very 'visible' institution in the immediate community and in the catchment area generally through its long history, first as a convalescent home for the poor, and then as a cancer treatment centre after the Second World War. Its name had become synonymous with the word 'cancer' in the surrounding community, and it had been regarded as a place of 'last resort' for those with 'no hope' of recovery, and with pain, suffering and death. These images are most vivid in the descriptions of patients whose own relatives were treated there 20 and 30 years previously. Modern treatment techniques have greatly improved the experience of radiotherapy however, and the centre had been steadily developing its modern service (both technologically and in terms of relations with patients and families). It had become a 'centre of excellence' with an international profile, and an important teaching facility. This change in image had not completely penetrated images of the centre held by the community at large, and the name of the centre still served as a diagnosis of cancer for prospective patients. Many patients interviewed said they felt the centre's name should be changed to distance it from its 'workhouse' past.

Much of the organization of staff and their work was geared to the maintenance of a unified, cheerful and informative service: patients were continually asked if they had any questions, and radiography and nursing staff were responsible for monitoring 'how patients were doing' as they moved through treatment. After assessment at a prescription clinic where patients were 'marked up' (tattooed) for treatment with the aid of a treatment simulator machine, they attended a weekly review clinic under a particular consultant. However, patients had the most contact with radiography and nursing staff, who were responsible for making referrals to the consultant if problems with treatment effects arose. Consultant staff and their registrars were almost entirely male, and radiography and nursing staff predominantly female, a pattern that has been typical of medical institutions generally.

The centre was in transition, shifting away from the image of the 'workhouse' and its historical reputation as a place of last resort for dying people condemned to pain and suffering, toward that of a modern, state-of-the-art cancer treatment centre offering efficient and friendly service. Changes in practice within it also reflected a broader transition in medicine generally, from the patriarchal, rigidly hierarchical organization with 'closed awareness' (Glaser and Strauss 1965) as the rule, to a more open, informative service ethic, in which lower status staff worked alongside high status medical professionals. (With regard to hierarchy it can be said that this specialist cancer treatment centre fell somewhere between the large, general acute-care institutions from which most patients are referred and the hospice in its organization: as in hospices, the emphasis in the centre was more on teamwork than hierarchy – although the hierarchy remained – with lower status staff in possession of a strong 'voice' in decision making and all aspects of the work of the centre.) This talk of transition within medicine generally is not to imply that a change in medical practice has occurred in its entirety, or that the more current ideal of 'open awareness' is achieved, but only that, at this point in the discursive shift away from old norms of practice, *both* the goals and practices of paternalistic medicine and those of a newer, more 'open' orientation apply.

City A centre radiotherapy patients

The centre offered treatment for a wide range of cancers, largely those of the head and neck, lung and breast. Thus patients in any of its waiting rooms differed greatly from one another in symptomatology depending on diagnosis and treatment site(s), and on the extensiveness of the disease. The waiting rooms always displayed a broad dimensional range of what 'cancer' can be and mean, and of who 'cancer patients' are. Patients spoke at length of the effect this contact had on their own struggle to define their experience. Sharing of personal stories and details of treatment was the expressed norm among patients, although the centre had printed material given to patients at the start of treatment advising them not to share such information. Patients were also warned verbally by staff not to discuss details of treatment with one another as their schedules progressed.

Radiotherapy at the centre

Radiotherapy treatment is both labour- and information-intensive in the planning phase, prior to the start of the treatment schedule itself. Planning involves defining the anatomic structures for treatment (the target volume) and the healthy tissues to be avoided (risk organs). Multiple target volumes may be defined for a particular patient, in cases where there is more than one tumour, or a likelihood of cancerous cells being present in several areas.

The appropriate dosage for each target volume, the number of treatments (or fractions) necessary, and the total treatment time must all be worked out, with the aid of imaging equipment and treatment simulators. The first step is a CT scan of the body area(s) in question, taken in the same position as during treatment, to provide the necessary anatomic information. It is then established how many radiation fields are appropriate, and their geometric position. Also, each treatment device (called a linear accelerator), even those from the same manufacturer, will differ, so the radiation field(s) must be measured for each one. In addition to the main schedule, shorter 'booster' schedules may be added to treat the tumour bed. A treatment simulator, a special x-ray device, is used to plan the actual administration of radiation. The patient lies in the treatment position(s) while x-ray images are taken of the radiation directions, including the planned field size(s) and form, and adjustments are made. The information is entered into the computers of each treatment machine. Radiotherapy itself takes about 5–15 minutes per person on average, given the time to position the patient as well as the actual treatment time. It can be much shorter, or much longer with the set-up taking up to an hour for an individual patient.

For most patients described here, several hours each day of treatment (weekdays for 4+ weeks on average) were involved in getting to treatment, receiving treatment and getting back home again, particularly if the person was reliant on ambulance transport. For many patients living outside the city, 5–7 hours a day were taken up in this way, most of which time was spent in an ambulance making pick-ups and drops at homes and hospitals to and from the clinic. Private transport and local residence cut down on time, but still, two to three hours could be taken up each day in the treatment process, and daily routines disrupted. Frequent machine break-downs and backlogs further slowed the process.

Radiotherapy treatment is a 'painless', even immaculate, process, unseen and unfelt, 'hi-tech' and computer-monitored. It does not remain immaculate however, as patients begin to experience the effects of accumulated treatments over time in the schedule, which can remain acute a long time after it is completed. Depending on the areas being treated and the extent of the treatment, patients can experience skin problems, sores, swelling and peeling (internally as well as externally), as well as diarrhoea, nausea, dizziness and enervation. Patients with cancers of the head, neck and upper respiratory tract experience the most serious 'side' effects, often producing problems with eating and taking in of fluids, and some may have to be hospitalized to prevent dehydration and malnutrition. Breast cancer patients report the fewest problems, experiencing reddened and irritated skin at the site of treatment.

The treatment work of the centre consisted in general of debilitating the disease in the newly diagnosed; minimizing progression in those with recurrences or advanced disease; preventing local recurrence; making surgery possible by shrinking tumour growth; and alleviating or minimizing symptoms caused by disease progression. For some patients, underlying this work would be the possibility of disease eradication, most likely as a result of a combination of modes of treatment.

Although the patients were newly diagnosed, 25 per cent were receiving palliative rather than radical treatment for advanced disease. There is a sense in which, while the 'public face' of the centre emphasized the eradication of cancer as the obvious central aim of cancer treatment (through emphasizing the 'success' of patients' surgery, for example, while neutralizing the prognostic issue and the limitations of treatment and medical knowledge), the actual work of the treatment centre was aimed at the *management* of cancer as a chronic illness. The (never overtly expressed) view of cancer treatment as primarily directed at 'cure' was pervasive both in patients' accounts of treatment and in discussions between the four consultants observed and their patients, and formed an intimate part of the 'service ideal' of the centre (Costain Schou 1993). This view was embodied in the seeming 'invisibility' of the prognosis issue in these encounters. Statements of prognosis, especially concerning specific statements about terminality and disease spread, appeared to be actively avoided. It emerged that prognostic information was withheld from several patients, or delivered in such an innocuous way that its implications were obscured (telling a breast cancer patient with newly discovered metastatic disease that a new 'spot' of cancer had been found on her spine and would require further treatment, for example). The elusiveness of the prognosis issue was seen to be a major feature of the 'ambiguous awareness' context of the treatment centre.

The term 'awareness context' appears in Glaser and Strauss's work on patients dying in American hospitals in the 1960s (Glaser and Strauss 1965). The term refers to the structures and processes involved in the production and management of awareness (of diagnosis, prognosis, implications of information, etc.). The awareness context forms a pervasive aspect of diagnosis and treatment contexts, ranging from 'closed' awareness where information, particularly that to do with prognosis and terminality, is withheld from patients, to 'open' awareness, where there are frank discussions between professionals and patients of all medical and treatment information as treatment progresses. While greater frankness about diagnosis and prognosis has been noted as a general trend in Britain and North America since the 1960s, the change in Britain has remained 'cautious and somewhat ambiguous', with an equivocal attitude to the question of awareness of threatening diagnoses and poor prognoses (Williams 1989: 204).

Far from being a passive experience, treatment involves a great deal of interpretive and practical work on the part of patients. From pre-diagnosis to post-treatment follow-up, patients must work at defining what treatment *is*, how they will deal with it, what information they need and how best to obtain it, and what choices to make in continuing to conduct their daily lives. Their definitions, interpretations and choices arise through their interaction with treatment professionals and other patients. Whatever is meant by a person's 'coping style' thus cannot be usefully separated from the individual's social reality. Psychosocial responses to treatment are also bound up with the pervasiveness of treatment in the lives of patients and their families, and with the social contexts comprising the treatment situation located within institutions involved in treatment work. In beginning this exploration of cancer patients' treatment experience, it will be useful to look at several aspects of the social context of City A treatment centre, through the accounts of several of its patients. These contextual features are also indicative of treatment as social interaction, a view of treatment that will be discussed in detail in the subsequent chapters. It should be noted here that while names and initials have been used to keep the sense of each excerpt as spoken by a real individual, these are entirely fictitious and bear no resemblance to the actual names of the persons involved. Some biographical information has also been included in order to provide a context for each excerpt and so that the reader will get a sense of 'who the speaker is'.

Locating treatment in context: the local world of City A treatment centre

> It's funny. You mention the word [centre's name] around this area, people will think you're on the scrap heap! [laughs] It's got a name of, you know they think, you only go there as a last resort, you know that people, have this ... because you only hear of really bad cases, they don't hear of all the good they do do they? It's strange, isn't it?
>
> (Meg, 50, housewife with breast cancer)

The image of the City A treatment centre as historically the 'end of the line' was vivid in many patients' descriptions of its community profile. Those who provided such descriptions were mostly in their sixties, and it was this group who expressed the most surprise over the centre's modern image, once they began treatment there. Here Ellie, 67, a retired catering assistant whose breast cancer was detected through routine screening, and her husband discuss a number of themes surrounding this contrast between then and now:

> ER: Yeah, I mean it ... *years* ago I mean it *was*, and I mean to go to [City A centre] *was* the end of the line. Because, before, I mean in *those* days =
>
> Husband: = Well, it's not as if, there was any treatment =
>
> ER: = There wasn't any treat ... well there was no *treat*ment either, there wasn't any treatment.

Husband: You were buried by the time you got to hospital, and *they* weren't quite sure and there wasn't any special in*su*rance . . .

ER: And there wasn't, and all this *after*-treatment was there?

Husband: You were nearly at death's *door* before you got to [the centre], so they hadn't a passing chance, of really getting you there to, uh . . . it's a miracle if they *did*, and if they did you'd got a very longwinded treatment, and very painful I would imagine. But *now*, with catching ladies, before it *hap*pens, they have 'em in and out and so on and, we shouldn't, have had her treatment, 10 or 15 years ago . . . if somebody's dropped in as a, you know, is it or isn't it 'cause they've found something themselves, and they get to hospital, well, I mean they just pass them along the *line* now to hospital. And of course at [City B], they haven't the facilities, I mean it's far too expensive and, 'cause they're specialized so they go, straight to [City A], so there's a hell of a lot better chance *now*, of coming out, you know their record used to be about, 10 per cent success 90 per cent failure of course, it's gone the other *way* now . . .

Here, the dismal past is contrasted with a very bright present, one described as owing to advances in treatment and detection. Both speakers exaggerate the contrast between the past and present (in the past there was 'no treatment', no detection and no chance, now women are 'caught' 'before it happens', and there is a 90 per cent 'success' rate).

This account gives voice to two important contextual features: the vivid image of the treatment centre in the community, and a view of modern cancer treatment echoed in many other patients' descriptions – that post-surgical treatment is 'just an insurance', or indeed, 'after-treatment'. At the same time Ellie's husband's emphasis on the 'success rate' of radiotherapy at the centre suggests conversely that such treatment is viewed much more seriously by both patients and staff. This discursive minimization/exaggeration of treatment's importance is a theme running through both professional and lay accounts of treatment, and is part of the construction of 'ambiguous awareness' which forms a major part of the social context of treatment.

One of the features of the centre which was described by many patients as most 'surprising' was the presence of 'younger' people being treated for cancer. Adam, 58, a retired textile worker with lung cancer, describes his impression of the radiotherapy clinic he attended:

AL: [City A centre] didn't affect me, no I thought it was a marvellous place. People round here's always . . . if [the centre] was mentioned we used to *shiver* you know. Not as much today but, I was surprised with the place when I went. *Very* much surprised.

KCS: What was it about it that surprised you?

AL: Well you know I thou . . . I'd thought it'd have been a dismal old place, and this that and the other but it was very bright. You saw, young ones walking round having chemotherapy and, smiles on their faces, and, I honestly *think*, in the waiting area that I used to wait in, I was surprisingly one of the oldest.

KCS: That was kind of an eye-opener.

AL: *Yeah* yeah yeah. Yes I would say I was one of the oldest. There was, you know, a few of my *age* but, in general there was a lot younger than me, which was surprising.

What descriptions like this one emphasize is the voiced contrast between previously held views, not just of the centre, but also of 'cancer' and 'cancer patients', with those based on patients' current contact with the clinic. Adam, who required help from neighbours and friends to drive him from his village to treatment at City A centre each weekday for several weeks, describes his friends' reactions of 'surprise' accompanying him into the waiting room:

AL: I think all but one of them went into the waiting room with me, one of them stopped in the car because he had his, telephone in the car you know he had a business.

KCS: Do you think they got anything out of being in the waiting room?

AL: They were very much sur*pri*sed, in *each* case, especially with what I mentioned before at how young some of them were. I mean in most of the cases they were touched by it, definitely. In all cases they were surprised *at* the appearance of the hospital. I mean there again, there was a few that took me there who were quite a bit older than me, and [the centre's name] were a dirty *word*, you know, going back years and years now.

A vivid image from patients' accounts is the unexpected overlap within the clinic of the 'outside' world and the world of the treatment centre. Accounts of waiting room experience contained repeated references to the variety of people present, a great percentage of whom were not patients at all, as described by Terry, 64, a retired electronics technician with cancer of the larynx, and his wife:

Wife: The people that brought their mums and dads, even *kids* in, playing outside they were, in one car park or in the field. The number of times we've come in and there's kids.

TL: Sometimes we've gone in, the waiting room was completely *full* and yet, there's probably only five *patients* among them! You know . . . just all friends that come in with them.

Wife: Yeah, my son and daughter's come here today, and that's their little girl and you know!

TL: Yeah, being up there isn't bad at all.

KCS: [the centre] by all accounts used to be a very depressing place.

TL: *Oh* it was, mention [the centre's name] and . . .

Wife: We used to take the kids when grandad were in.

TL: They used to play on the grass outside.

Wife: It was difficult. Grandad used to sit in the, where the doors were and then watch me and the kids play, and Terry would go and sit in for a half hour and then, *he*'d go out to the kids and *I*'d go and sit for a while. We had to sit out with the children, they couldn't go *in*, always outside.

Here, a rich (if potentially cumbersome!) community presence is described, with whole families accompanying patients to treatment. This view is contrasted in the account with a vignette from what might be called this couple's 'family illness past' (visiting Grandad at the centre), in which an image of the centre's 'closed awareness' past is evoked. The historical cancer hospital, rigidly cut off from the surrounding community through fear (of the disease, the institution itself, and its work) is transformed in these accounts into the modern treatment centre, open to the 'well' community, young and old alike.

Changing views of cancer and treatment

The perspectives of the centre constructed by patients were linked to accounts of changed perspectives of treatment and of 'cancer'. Phil, 58, a bait farm worker forced to retire after losing a leg in an accident, was receiving palliative radiotherapy for lung cancer. Here he recalls a friend's death from cancer at a time when 'going in' to hospital for treatment often meant never coming out again:

PH: I realize now that today we've improved a lot I mean, when you think back. I mean I know of at least three people who died of cancer and there wasn't a thing they could do *for* them and, they were only young people like. One of them in particular was a chap, a member of a club I'm in, the last 30-odd years. He were 42 years old, never drank hardly never smoked in his life, and they had him in the infirmary with pains in his back and we was going visiting and most of the lads I knew used to visit him, and he never come out of the infirmary. He just laid there and wasted away and died. There wasn't anything they could do, and they didn't have any of these treatments and that then and so, you know. Probably the same thing would have happened to me in the . . . if it had been back to those days you know that they couldn't have done anything for me but I mean all they had was tablets, they didn't have any, radiotherapy or chemotherapy or anything like that you know.

Radiotherapy and chemotherapy have been in use since the middle and late nineteenth century respectively (Horwich and Duchesne 1988), but today they are common modes of treatment, even in cases of advanced and terminal disease. In fact, the greatest strides in cancer treatment generally have been made in palliation, or the management of symptoms and disease spread in advanced cancer, rather than in increased 'cure' rates for most cancers. Phil, who had earlier expressed his awareness of his poor prognosis, describes a contrast between his experience in the present, and 'those days' in the past when 'they couldn't have done anything for me', and 'treatment' would have consisted of 'tablets' and dying in hospital.

Many patients' accounts emphasized treatment as a learning experience during which they had come to see it in a more complex light, despite the lack of certainty surrounding their own outcomes. Adam, who was undergoing a radical six-week course of radiotherapy for inoperable lung cancer, describes a changed perspective in this excerpt:

> AL: The only thing positive that's come out of [having cancer] from *my* point of view is that I know a great deal more *about* it than what I did. As I say, [the centre's name] were a dirty word, and that sort of thing. The positive thing that's come out of it, is [the centre] can do you *good*. And, it might make you poorly first, but nevertheless, you know it can do you good. I'm more positive thinking now that, cancer isn't the be-all and end-all of life. You know, you can get over it.

At the time of his treatment, there was a *Panorama*[4] programme on regional disparities in cancer treatment in Britain that many patients described watching with great interest. Adam had been a nurse for a short time in his youth before leaving the health service to take a better paid job as a textile worker, and expressed great interest in 'anything to do with medical matters'. The *Panorama* documentary seemed to have cast his situation in a new light by placing the local treatment centre in a national context:

> AL: It was that programme on telly about cancer the other night. It didn't bother me watching it, where a lot of people it *would*. I were quite interested in it. It was basically how, treatment compared from area to area. I mean I'm so . . . from *my* point of view and seeing that, I thought how lucky I was to be in the [City A] regional area, where there was this radiotherapy and, and that sort of thing. I think in some areas, in Scotland etc. that, there's nowhere *near* any cancer research hospitals or, you've far less chance of uh, surviving.

Adam describes himself as 'lucky' to receive treatment at a research institution that stands out favourably in a national context of variable access to technology and expertise in cancer treatment. Rachael, 41, a part-time schoolteacher with breast cancer who had seen the same programme, also describes herself as fortunate:

> RS: There *was* actually a programme on *Panorama*, while I was having my, radiotherapy, about breast cancer, and different, approaches to treatments, and how hit and miss the treatment was, regarding as to where you *lived*, and what hospitals you were treated in and I felt really *lucky*, that I was treated in a specialist hospital, whereas, there were people on there that, you know were just treated in a normal general hospital and they weren't getting the, uh, specialized treatment that I feel *I* got. So I felt lucky in that respect.

The discovery that modern cancer treatment is not a commonplace throughout Britain placed the City A treatment centre in a national context as a 'specialist hospital' offering 'specialized treatment'. The increased visibility in the media of cancer treatment, and the whole issue of management of health service resources, was widely commented upon by the patients, clearly forming part of the social context of their treatment experiences.

Consistent treatment by individuals

Dan, 76, a retired merchant seaman with cancer of the bladder, describes his experiences as an in-patient receiving palliative radiotherapy:

> DG: My wife's father, he had this. He had a prostate and, he had treatment at [the centre] which, going back eight to nine years ago, but it seems to be, you know a different hospital now to what it was *then* you know.
>
> KCS: In what way?
>
> DG: In a good way... well it were very very austere you know, it was a *hos*pital, heh heh! You know! Whereas now it, it seems to be more, more like a *home*. I mean the staff are, they come round, and they've all got their badges with their names on and, a little dark girl there came in, she was a sister. And she looked up above me bed she says, Daniel G, I says yeah, she says what do you want calling Mr G? Oh Dan I says, Dan'll do me. OK she says, my name's Lily. And uh, everything seemed, you know, *home*y and, you know different to the old cold idea of, you're here to get done, or... oh it seemed different altogether. I have no compunction about going in.

Whereas once the centre was an 'austere . . . *hos*pital', now it is a 'home', and this change is linked here to the speaker's contact with 'staff', all of whom are identified as individuals via name badges. Dan illustrates his account with specific reference to one encounter with one staff member very different from himself ('a little dark girl'). Discovering connections between himself and other staff, and developing real relationships with several, was also described as central to his avowed changed view of the centre:

DG: They've a big place up at [the centre], and loads of students round. I felt quite at home [there] because, two of the lasses . . . whenever you go for this treatment there's about four nurses, to put you on and pull you, twist you and turn you . . . they came from *Scot*land, Scots lassies, and they were very very nice.

Wife: And when you were *in*, the ambulance ladies all went to see him every day when he was in.

DG: The girls that used to pick me up here and take me, and then bring me back. But when I was in for the week, as soon as they'd got in and got their patients off they'd come straight up to the ward and have a drink of coffee with me. Other times, I would get dressed, walk down to the cafe and have a coffee with them, and both of them . . . there was two, Joanne and Gail, and they both came to see me, waiting for the other patients to have their treatment.

Although the centre is a 'big' and very busy teaching facility, its day-to-day 'business' *is* the social contact between patients and staff described here. Details that comprise consistency in treatment experience – always seeing the same individuals during treatment, learning first names of staff members, being able to visit in the coffee shop – also distinguish treatment as social interaction. Betty, 44, a retired Chief WREN with breast cancer who was accompanied to treatment by her mother, describes consistency in contact with treatment staff and among patients:

KCS: How many other people do you see usually, you see the radiographers of course =

BG: = At [the centre] I mean you'd have, four radiographers, all the same ones every day, so you get to know them, and chat to the same women every day. Then the patients, and then once a week I'd see the three nurses, and either Dr X or his, Indian friend wish I knew what his *name* was 'cause I mean I see him all the *time* you know. And then we usually go upstairs and have a cup of tea, see the same people up there and [laughs slightly] it's amazing the people I mean, people there from [City B], and we didn't *realize*, you know all the people from [several villages near City A] all *over* the place, all discussing their, you know, what the traffic was like in the morning and that . . . it is it's like it was a little family, a little, you know just generally chatting, before you go and a cup of tea afterwards, puts you in a right frame of *mind*.

The daily 'flow' of the clinic, comprised of consistent contact with radiographers and weekly consultations with consultants and registrars, as well as the diversity of other patients and family members, seemed to give the weekly experience of radiotherapy a secure rhythm for many patients. Betty describes the importance of this security:

KCS: So you get to know people?

BG: Yes, yes. Which is *good.* 'Cause it's painless, and you're seeing the same people and conversation is not *stilted* and it's so free and I think that puts you at ease as well. I mean, it's trying to take the worry away from something you can't, afford, to let anything else into a stressful situation. It gets rid of all the dread, the, stress, and I found at [the centre], everywhere you'd been, if you went somewhere, you know you were *tak*en there, everybody *knew*, what every other department was doing, and what . . . you've got to go in so-and-so, right, your marks came off, OK we'll replace all the marks. I remember I'd washed off my marks in the bath one night. Well, I had to go back on the simulator again. They said, don't worry, you know. And then when I went down, the simulator knew I was coming you know, and we had a little joke, about, serves you right! You know, *back* on the simulator again, this will teach you to scrub too hard in the bath, and this kind of thing. I think it's *good*, everybody knew, where you were, and why you were *there*.

Betty here describes a connected service, with good coordination between departments. Her emphasis that patients 'cannot afford to let anything else' of an anxiety-producing nature into what is already a 'stressful situation' evokes another aspect of the social experience of treatment: the task of management of the resources used and drawn upon in treatment, in the patient's case, primarily those of time, energy and attention. In the social context of treatment, professionals are responsible for managing and coordinating their work in such a way that the centre's institutional resources are well-used and conserved. However, their management work must also see that patients' personal resources are not squandered. It will be argued in this book that such resources, ranging from money, time and expertise to perhaps more abstract notions of energy and attention, are the medium through which both personal identity and the social experience of treatment are constructed and maintained.

Many patients described chaotic diagnostic experiences in the large general hospitals to which they had usually been referred before coming to the centre for treatment. The 'everydayness' of the centre, with its friendly atmosphere and dependable care, seemed to form the foundation for the social contact among patients there, and between patients and staff.

The social world of the clinic

The single most distinguishing feature of the centre was the diversity of people in its clinic waiting rooms. At any given point in the day, these rooms contained people of all age groups, both sexes, different social classes, different diagnoses and prognoses, from different towns and villages, both cancer patients and non-cancer patients. This diversity was vividly and spontaneously described in patients' accounts of treatment, as in Phil's below:

> PH: Do you know they . . . a lot of people what I, I met at the clinic were from outside the [City A] area. It's surprising how far people come from. Actually, this last time I went, there was a chappy came in and he was really jazzed up, he wasn't a young man he was getting on. He had on really jazzy clothes you know, he had on a sweater with the name of a club in America. I started talking to him and it turned out that for 30 years he's worked in America, and he's come back here and bought himself a house, they're retired now . . . There was a lot of people from the place I come from [near City B] I could tell from the way they spoke. And in particular, there was this chappy, he was the same as me he had *lung* cancer. And I asked how he was doing, and he says well, he says they told me I was going to die in a month and that were two ruddy *year* ago! [laughs]

Other patients were arguably the most significant contextual feature of the treatment centre for people undergoing treatment there. Although waiting room experience has been depicted in the literature as anxiety-producing (Fallowfield and Clark 1991), seeing that 'there's always someone worse off than you' was routinely described as comforting rather than depressing, despite patients' expressed initial fears about 'what really ill' people would look like. Any waiting room observer will see a cross-section of 'what really does go on', as one long-time patient commented, and will hear many frank conversations during an hourly wait. The 'geography of illness' that emerged was described as surprising by patients in interviews, such as Sam, 66, a retired salesman with melanoma:

> SM: I think people there like it actually, you know sort of chatting, when you're in the waiting room. You just visit, and they come

from all over the place you know. And, you think it's just you in your district and there isn't because, when you get on the ambulance you find there's someone else. And, you know, they were from [names several cities and towns] all over the place you know, you don't know until you get talking to them, but it's nice to *get* talking and find out where people come from.

There was much talk amongst patients (and talk about talk in interviews) about treatment, prognosis, diagnostic experiences, practical problems, side effects, the weather, hobbies – indeed as varied a list of topics as any divergent group of people forced by circumstances to come together for several hours a day can find to discuss. Some of this talk was intimate, about advanced disease, poor prognoses and recurrences – first-time diagnosis patients often found themselves in conversation with long-term cancer survivors. Alice, 50, a soft furnishings store owner with breast cancer, describes such a meeting:

AW: Everybody wants to help each other because I s'pose they all knew they were in the same *boat*. I met one chap who had cancer of the *face* and he's been, suffering, for 11 *years*, and, he lost one eye. He's got plastic surgery halfway down his head all the way down his face at one side. It had got into the *bone*, behind his, other eye or somewhere near his other eye and he had to have radium, for the first time, to see if they could arrest it. I think the first thing they ever told him was, he would lose his *sight*, and I never heard that man complain, went with him every day for two and a half weeks and he said, I feel so sorry for the surgeon he said, he's battled with me for 11 years. And, I said you must have had a lot of pain he said *oh* no the drugs are very good you know. So positive in his thinking. You know that they *help* you along. There's no *way* you're going to give in to negative thought when you're talking to people like *that* because, all the rest of the time he was so *in*teresting to talk to.

In the waiting room, advanced illness, the ravages of treatment, survivorship and the many faces of 'cancer' as a collection of different chronic illnesses are visible on a daily basis. Contact with other patients seemed to have had a dimensionalizing effect on individuals' expressed views of their illness: a spectrum of cancer diagnoses/prognoses and cancer patients had replaced what for most people was limited or no experience with either.

Many patients described their initial fears about 'what it was going to be *like*' in terms of how 'depressing' the centre and its patients were going to be, and whether treatment was going to be a daily reminder of suffering and death. These fears seemed to have been dispelled after the start of treatment schedules. Alice points out both the negative and positive aspects of the presence of many other patients there:

> AW: I *think* it's a daunting place, [the centre], it's an old-fashioned hospital it's a bit depressing. There are so many people, coming and going all the time there are *so* many people, that – with the *ill*ness, I mean – you just, just can't imagine . . . of course you don't have far to look for faces, somebody a lot worse off than yourself. And you meet some, very *sweet* people, as you chat to them. I don't think I spoke to one person that hadn't, come to terms with what was happening or, you just never come across negativity. I didn't anyway.

The centre was in a partially-renovated state at the time interviews with these patients took place, with some waiting and treatment areas bright and modern, including carpeting, recessed lighting and fishtanks, and the rest drab and institutional, unchanged since the 1960s. But the presence of 'so many people' with cancer is a potentially overwhelming feature of a large treatment centre, and it is this concern that the centre staff cited as the reason for the written and verbal warnings to patients not to share details of their treatment or illness with one another. These warnings were acknowledged by patients, but every interview was replete with accounts of encounters with other patients and their families in the waiting rooms and centre coffee shop. Meg, 50, a housewife with breast cancer, describes making a contact at the clinic despite her concern for privacy:

> MG: They [other patients] are all very chatty and, and I think it's nice if you can talk to somebody who, you know, tells you what they're going through. There is one woman, well like me, and I, I was sur*prise*d because, you see I, how do you say, I'm a bit, a bit private I'd say, and I don't like people to know my business, so at first I wouldn't tell anybody, and of course I met a lady there who is exactly the *same*, she doesn't want her friends to know. I mean the close friends yes they know, but people who I just say hello to and that, I mean you don't go around telling everybody, what you've got.

Many patients were working to prevent too much disclosure of their situations outside the centre, but described finding a 'comfort level' of sharing within it. Hillary, 63, a housewife with breast cancer, described her discomfort at the presence of a volunteer counsellor who occasionally used the waiting room to contact and speak with breast cancer patients. This lack of privacy (the centre did not have a designated counselling room at this time) was cited by several women as their reason for not wanting to meet with the counsellor. Hillary describes finding another patient with whom she did feel comfortable, in the same waiting room:

HB: And then there's an*oth*er lady who I got more friendly with. I
don't know *her* well either but she's the sort of person, I felt
I would talk to *more*, and, she didn't have what I've got but she
had a cancer you know, so. No, I don't mind talking to people,
and you know I haven't, I haven't talked to, you know swap
notes with patients like they say you're not supposed to do.

Patients described finding their own levels of interaction in the waiting
room, despite the staff position against sharing treatment and illness details between patients.

From 'dirty word' to 'little world': the modern treatment centre

Martha, 48, a secretary with breast cancer, describes the social context of
the treatment centre as separate from the 'normal world':

MF: It's very open there's no uh, problem . . . that is *one* thing that,
I mean I'm going, I say you're going to *miss*, I mean *they've*
come out with it well, I have cancer you have cancer, what do
you have you have cancer, yes, I mean you don't, in everyday
conversation you s— this is . . . this is not going to happen, you
know. Once I'm back in the normal world again.

KCS: So that will be a bit of a shock =

MF: = Well I think you've got to, yes, yes. You're not going to discuss it with everyone that's for sure. And, it's a . . . it's a different really *world* we're, at the *m*oment I mean we're more or less
living in that little world of ambulance, [the centre], home, you
know, and that's three weeks there, that's finished and, I think
there's support. You, you feel there is some support, and then if
you've got a worry, you can discuss it when you go there, but
when, once we've finished it I think we're going to be on our
own rather.

In patients' accounts, the comforting 'little world' of the centre was
often drawn in contrast to the 'outside' world, largely in terms of the easy
waiting room contact with other patients, and the disclosure to others this
contact provided of problems and details of treatment and illness. Alice
describes another, more existential image of contrast between the world of
the centre and that outside it:

AW: Oh, everybody's so chatty, you know it's, a little bit of a different
world, to what you ever, *touch* on, especially when you're in the
rat race and there's so much *greed* that it's pathetic. The rest
of the time, it makes you wonder what you've been *do*ing with
your life . . . it just opens your mind up to a different *world*, and

makes you wonder what you've been doing when, I mean, from nurses to doctors to what *ever*. They all seem to have a, better *cause* than I've given myself to . . . You just meet so *many* people – unless you're in an involvement – that just absolutely live for materialism. But I've never known where to go from *there*, to find involvement with people that don't think that way, and suddenly I was thrown into it, and I found it quite stimulating.

Alice, who ran her own soft furnishings business, describes a new world of meaning in the treatment centre with apparently different values to those she encountered in the business world in which she moved. The treatment centre as a social world was described at times in patients' accounts as operating according to different 'rules' from that outside it, in that it was a more 'open' world, in which the familiar social barriers common in the general social context no longer applied, at least not as rigidly. Distinctions of geography, accent, class, gender and age were described as mattering less within the treatment context, while similarities with other patients, medical or personal, seemed to suggest that cancer patients are also 'normal people', like oneself. The clinic as a source of supportive interactions with others in treatment in an egalitarian atmosphere was a major theme in patients' accounts, such as Betty's below:

> BG: It's been *very* helpful because you, you know like your first day there, you haven't got a *clue* I mean, just report to outpatients. You haven't got a clue what it was going to be *like* you know. As the days progress, you know, and you *knew* people there and start talking, you're like a big happy family. When you finish you know, all the people say, 'Oh it's my last day, all the best, may see you around', something like that. 'Oh how many *more* have you got to go, oh well there you are.' It was *great*, you know, and it was good for mum as well. I mean whilst I was in having me treatment, she'd be there chatting away and, 'Oh Mrs So-and-so's having so-and-so', and, someone's, you know no one's sat looking at each other like you do on a British Rail train or something like that, or nobody's where nobody *says* anything I mean. No, it was great, I wonder why. You're all there, you know you want to know, a bit more the next *day*, 'cause you're all there for the same thing, and there's no airs and graces. Normal people having the same thing, it's an equal thing each to you all.

Conversation at the centre was described as freer than that between strangers in the world outside the centre and often of a remarkably intimate nature. Betty's account emphasizes the communication between patients as both ordinary (about the mundane details of the treatment calendar) and extraordinary, in that there is contact distinctly different from that which takes place between strangers outside the centre, in the general social context. The image of social equality of patients in treatment at the same centre emerged strongly from such accounts.

Summary

This chapter has introduced some problems with the depiction of treatment experience in the psychosocial oncology literature, and introduced an alternative view of treatment as social interaction. Several contextual features of a particular treatment institution, as described in patients' accounts and authors' observations, have been highlighted. The depiction of 'treatment' in the literature as a neutral, 'antiseptic' process to which individuals react in idiosyncratic ways locates problems and concerns in treatment *in* the treated individual, rather than in the process of treatment itself. This individualism is a feature of both biomedical models of treatment, and the dominant cognitivism of psychosocial oncology.

But 'treatment' consists in social interaction; it is through interaction between individuals and groups within specific contexts that people become patients and experience treatment; therefore it is important to examine such contexts carefully. City A treatment centre emerged in patients' accounts as a highly 'visible' social context (for both cancer patients and members of the 'well' community in a broad geographical area), not an anonymous institution. The centre's 'closed awareness' past continued to be voiced alongside evidence of its more 'open' (but not uncomplicated) modern orientation as a 'state of the art' treatment centre. The centre formed part of a national context of health care and cancer treatment, plagued by serious issues of resources management and distribution. The centre was an informal forum for contact between disparate groups of people, both cancer patients and non-patients, laypeople and health professionals, in which the effects of treatment and disease, survivorship, terminal illness and death from cancer were regularly visible. Here, 'social support' can be seen as a main activity of the centre, in one respect its actual biomedical treatment work forming a comparatively small part of the sum of the 'total arc of work' performed in it (Corbin and Strauss 1988). In this social context, a dimensional range of what 'cancer' can be and mean, and of what a 'cancer patient' is, is readily apparent.

In Chapters 3, 4 and 5 the treatment centre described here continues to provide the context for our exploration of treatment experience and quality of life in treatment. Diagnosis and the early illness calendar lead into setting up and preparing for the treatment calendar. After this phase, the treatment calendar itself dominates the lives of patients. These phases of the treatment experience are explored in the following three chapters.

Notes

1 All patients attended City A centre for treatment prescription and reviews, and for radiotherapy. Some patients attended City B hospital for chemotherapy because they lived in or near City B. However, City A centre is the primary treatment context for all patients described in this book.
2 The interviews were analysed as transcribed texts, proceeding from 'open coding', during which relevant concepts, images, themes and patterns within and between interviews were noted down, through to axial and selective coding, during which a conceptual framework was developed. The analysis involves close reading and rereading of the interview material throughout the data collection process, with earlier interviews suggesting new directions for subsequent ones, and so forth. For a more complete description of the methodology, see Appendix.
3 The centre is now scheduled for closure, following relocation of treatment services for cancer patients to a large hospital in City A.
4 *Panorama* is an investigative current affairs programme on BBC television.

3 | Diagnosis and the early illness calendar

In this chapter, we introduce several key concepts in our analysis of patients' accounts of treatment experience. These ideas are central to our depiction in this book of treatment and quality of life as *social* and socially constructed. We then move on to describe and discuss the *early illness calendar*, which begins with the diagnostic period and provides the context for the treatment calendar(s).

The calendar as central analytic construction

Our analysis in this chapter of accounts of early treatment experience for a first-time diagnosis of cancer makes use of the notion of the calendar. A calendar can be defined as any plan involving the ordering of time, and the notion of stages to be negotiated at specific times/places along a trajectory. It is an essentially linear mode of structuring and organizing all aspects of living, pervasive in the discourses of Western cultures.[1] The individual illness and treatment calendars of patients are experienced in a context of individuals' personal and life calendars, and of those calendars that punctuate both personal and community life and that are tied to the 'calendar year'.

This latter type of calendar refers to the actual organization of time into days, weeks and months, and to specific points within the organization, like bank holidays and Christmas, that serve as markers of a general cultural and communal context. For example, Jewish people in Britain will still experience Christmas as a calendar event even though they do not experience it as a religious occasion or as involving required rituals, like present-giving and so forth.

Some calendars have the status of what Schutz and Luckman (1974) call 'social structures of relevance', embodying goals, motivations and limitations experienced by each individual as part of a common social context. Whether or not one rejects traditional life calendar goals such as marriage and children, particularly before a certain age is reached, is not the point. These 'goals' still exist as social norms among some groups of people, while they represent deviation to others. They are thus identifiable as 'objects of the life calendar'. Calendars and the actions of calendar construction and calendar keeping are a manifestation of 'the and so forth idealization' (Schutz and Luckman 1974), articulated by Schutz as the trust that

> the world as it has been known by me up until now will continue further and that consequently the stock of knowledge obtained from my fellow-men and formed from my own experiences will continue to preserve its fundamental validity.
>
> (Schutz and Luckman 1974: 7)

Calendars represent such a 'stock of knowledge' and the assurance is implicit within their construction and use that the world will continue in a relatively predictable manner. Within the experience of chronic illness, predictability based on previous, pre-diagnosis experience is threatened. At the same time, actions involved in calendar-keeping become more complicated and crucial in the struggle to manage life within the new dictates of the illness calendar. In the illness and treatment calendars, predictability has to be continually reconstructed and a greater degree of unpredictability tolerated as illness and treatment cause frequent disruptions to calendar-keeping.

In Schutz and Luckman's phenomenology, the lifeword is the province above all of practice and action. In daily life, acts are 'components within a higher-order system of plans: for a specific province within the lifeworld, for the day, for the year, for work and leisure – which in turn have their place in a more or less determined life-plan' (1974: 19). We have conceptualized this system of plans in terms of several broad types of calendars to be discussed further in the present chapter and in those that follow: the 'personal' or 'private' calendar, the life calendar, the illness calendar and the treatment calendar.

Our notion of the 'personal' and 'private' calendar incorporates the schedules of the daily life of the individual, which are comprised of various acts, responsibilities, goals and so forth. At a deeper level though, we also take on board Sacks's notion of the private calendar as composed of 'ways of building up, in deep and repetitive ways, the relevance of "you"' (Sacks 1989: 212). Sacks was referring to the private calendars constructed between people in specific close relationships (such as marriage) that serve as a means of locating both private events within the relationship but also events in the world in general by reference to the relationship. For example, an event of significance in the relationship, like an anniversary, might serve to locate an event of significance for the general calendar, like a national election date. When the 'we' of the private calendar ends, so does this calendar, while 'everybody else's' calendar goes on. In our use of this term, the private calendar is a personal calendar, one which encompasses specific close relationships and their calendars as well as others relating to personal identity (although it must be noted that all calendars contribute to personal identity). Also encompassed by the personal calendar are the demands of the daily 'lifeworld' of the individual, demands which will also overlap with and involve the personal calendars of other people. The personal calendar is thus distinct from, although interacting with, the general socio-cultural calendar and the calendar year, and is subsumed by the life calendar of the individual.

As noted earlier, a cancer diagnosis causes huge disruptions both in the life calendars of individuals and in their day-to-day personal calendars. It also introduces new calendars of illness and treatment which initially dominate the personal and life calendars of patients. 'Coping' and coming to terms with the diagnosis and treatment can be conceptualized as negotiation and the management of these new calendars, as well as the task of dealing with the larger, more existential issues of the future, of life and death, contained in the life calendar and thrown into relief by a cancer diagnosis. The notion of the many calendars through which we make sense of experience and the practical demands it brings allows us to speak of both the personal and social aspects of this experience in a more fluid way, showing them to be graphically interconnected at all times.

The social nature of 'quality of life' is revealed in the arenas of experience demarcated by illness and treatment calendars. Professionals in charge of the treatment calendar have an area of work distinct from 'giving' a diagnosis or 'administering' treatment – namely, that of treatment calendar management. This management work is intimately bound up with the general culture of biomedicine and the unique cultures of individual medical institutions, and with the actions of individual professionals within these social contexts. Such work is also bound up with political and resources agendas of the institutional and larger social contexts involved. Illness and treatment calendar management directly involve social aspects of health care and treatment experience that remain largely unaddressed in the quality of life literature, and yet can be seen to impact greatly on patients' experienced 'quality of life' as this is constructed in interview accounts of treatment experience. Within our analysis, the 'experience of illness' is seen as ultimately bound up with the experience of illness calendar and treatment calendar management.

Illness and treatment trajectories and calendars

A trajectory is also time-bound, but is intended here to mean a projection, whereas the calendar is a concrete plan (or composed of such plans, like schedules). The distinction here between projected and concrete illness and treatment plans is developed by Corbin and Strauss (1988) who discuss 'illness trajectories' in terms of 'trajectory projections' and 'trajectory plans'. In our framework, the treatment *calendar* is the concrete plan, or manifestation of the projection, or treatment *trajectory*. Trajectories are also templates for calendars. A trajectory formulation in diagnosis and treatment is based on ideas about what might/could/should happen at different points in an experience over time, based on probability and the assessment of contextual features. A calendar, on the other hand, is based on what *will* happen at certain points along a trajectory projection (not excluding the fact that calendar points can be subject to frequent disruption). As the trajectory projection changes, so does the calendar.[2] Yoshida (1993) advocates the term 'illness trajectory' (as a 'pendulum', with both forward and backward movement possible within it) to describe illness experience, rather than the more linear and orderly 'career'. Our trajectory projections are linear (as they are the templates for calendars), but interrupted and changed frequently as new information becomes available, or the disease course changes.

Treatment trajectories exist in the minds of treatment planners and managers – they are *not* exposed to patients directly (except in rare instances) but are instead intuited by patients and hinted at by practitioners. Treatment calendars on the other hand are made known in varying degrees to patients (otherwise they could not be implemented) and can be discussed by patients and others by virtue of their 'public' nature. They are subject to change, however, as the agent/manager sees the disease trajectory as changed, and thus adjusts the treatment trajectory accordingly, following it through the implementation of a new treatment calendar. Patients have their own trajectory ideas of course, and these are developed through the tackling of various definitional tasks and strategies.

Corbin and Strauss (1988) are concerned with the management of varied kinds of work in the management of chronic illness by patients at home. They point to three kinds of work facing patients and their families: illness-related, biographical, and everyday-life work. We have conceptualized these three arenas of work in terms of the organization of time. In this framework, the illness-related work arena is defined by the illness and treatment calendars, the biographical work arena by the life calendar, and the everyday-life work arena by the personal or private calendar. Of course, all of these contexts overlap: illness and treatment-related work becomes a main feature of the private or personal calendar for example, and biographical work must be carried out and threats to it dealt with within each context. As mentioned in Chapter 2, Corbin and Strauss (1988: 90–1) call the above lines of work the 'total arc of work to be accomplished over any specific period of time'. The notion of illness and treatment as involving work to be done within a time frame necessitates a focus on resources, those of time, energy, money, space, and others in a variety of contexts.

Different tasks at different stages of trajectory (or here, calendar) management require different resources, and Corbin and Strauss point out that there is competition for resources between the three lines of work.

Diagnosis and the beginning of treatment for cancer

The central feature of this period is the interconnected nature of diagnosis and early treatment procedures and treatment calendar planning and implementation. The *illness calendar* begins with the diagnostic period and is the immediate context within which all subsequent treatment and consultations take place. In a sense it never really comes to an end – the patient will always be subject to reviews and semi-annual checks after treatment is completed. It is often instigated by the experience of physical instability (which becomes 'symptoms' through diagnosis), and begins properly once a consultation is made with a medical professional. The central issue in the early illness calendar is diagnosis and treatment set-up; within the individual treatment calendars and the later illness calendar, the key issues are prognosis, and living with the effects of treatment and the changed life context instigated by illness and treatment.

We will refer to the illness and treatment calendars separately, but in fact the illness calendar, consisting of all consultations, appointments, checks, reviews etc. to do with the illness, is the context for the individual treatment calendars experienced by each patient. *Treatment calendars* are calendars for the discrete courses of treatment given to each patient. There will be a separate calendar for a course of radiotherapy, and one for a course of chemotherapy for the same patient, for example. These discrete calendars, along with the other consultations and appointments the patient must keep, such as those for prescription and follow-up, make up the illness calendar in its entirety.

Newly-diagnosed patients are forced to deal with the sudden disruption, both actual and threatened, of their life calendars. 'Life calendars' subsume future plans, plans related to the attaining of goals, work achievements, relationships, and the calendar of day-to day living. For the patient, the treatment calendar is the 'lived' treatment plan or trajectory, while the trajectory itself is in the hands of treatment managers and agents. The gap between the treatment calendar and the trajectory plan represents an imposing awareness gap for the patient and family members or close others. The treatment calendar is composed of one or more schedules of treatment, and while it is made known to the patient, the reasoning behind it rarely is. Health care professionals are seen here as agents of the treatment calendar, and as treatment calendar managers. When they do this job well, they are able to help provide a more liveable context for their patients in treatment and in the illness calendar as a whole.

Contextual features of the diagnostic process

The cancer diagnostic course often resembles an obstacle course rather more than it does a neat, straight line. Accounts of diagnosis in the literature tend to give the impression of 'diagnosis' as consisting of carefully managed, single conversations in private settings, including presentation of a treatment rationale and prognostic information, held (presumably) after a linear process of 'symptoms' → consultation → referral → tests → confirmation of cancer (although typically, little information is given about the process of arriving at the diagnosis).

The considerable medical ambiguity surrounding cancer diagnosis, staging and treatment planning is one reason for complex and, at times, chaotic diagnostic courses. Diagnosis can involve many tests, many of which have to be repeated. Complexity arises when there are several different types of professional involved, different hospital departments and even different institutions. Also, early treatment and diagnosis often go hand-in-hand, with patients having tumours or body parts removed, and beginning chemotherapy. Diagnosis and prognosis are compounded issues, as are diagnosis and treatment calendar planning. Establishing operability (which has a direct bearing on prognosis) and deciding the appropriate treatment trajectory are part of becoming diagnosed. Diagnostic information often comes in piecemeal, as test results are returned and initial surgery performed. This information can be conflicting and hard to interpret, and there can be delays and mix-ups emanating from mislaid results or poor communication between departments and professionals.

An earlier complicating factor involves the initial consultation which begins the cancer illness calendar. Patients consult because they experience physical instability that troubles them enough to seek a doctor's help – they do not necessarily experience 'symptoms' of cancer *per se*. Their initial instability must first be defined as 'serious' or 'suspicious' if they are to be diagnosed with cancer. Many cancer patients experience long delays in becoming diagnosed at this stage, because their 'symptoms' are thought to relate to an acute illness or condition, perhaps treatable with antibiotics, or to an existing chronic condition, like heart disease.

Alternatively, there may be no experience of instability, with the diagnostic process begun as a result of routine screening, such as a mammogram, or by chance at a general 'check-up', or while consulting for something minor. On the other hand, diagnosis for cancer may begin as a physical crisis (a sudden, searing pain, or attack of breathlessness for example) that descends 'out of the blue' and that initiates a complex hospital illness calendar. People may struggle for a long time with instability before initial consultation. Becoming committed to a complex illness calendar is intimidating, and the person may intuitively avoid seeing instability as 'serious' or 'suspicious' for this reason. Loss of work time and pay is a major issue

---

Box 3.1: *Disruptions in the illness and treatment calendars* – *Gerald's case*

It is apparent from this discussion that the treatment calendar can be prey to a variety of delays and set-backs that will have an impact on how it is perceived and experienced by the patient. It will be useful for the purposes of summary to look at the details of Gerald's early illness and treatment calendars, verified through his medical records and diary record of the events, as they contain many types of complication, both organic and institutional, that can befall diagnosis and treatment calendar set-up. His was the most extreme case, but almost all the patients interviewed had dealt with multiple and quite complex treatment calendar problems at one stage or another.

Gerald, 58, a retired engineer with lung cancer, presented to his GP the Friday before Christmas, having coughed up blood on the Thursday night. He was immediately sent to a local hospital for an x-ray which was processed promptly and which revealed that the upper lobe of his right lung had collapsed. Gerald and his wife were due to go away until after the New Year, so the GP decided to refer him for a bronchoscopy after the holiday.

1 After Gerald returned from his holiday, he received a letter from the consultant who was to do the bronchoscopy, giving him an appointment for the procedure itself (without which he would have had to attend twice, once for assessment and once for the bronchoscopy), because the clinic schedule had been disrupted by the holidays, and there was a backlog to clear.

2 The weekend before Gerald's appointment, he broke out in shingles around his mouth which prohibited the bronchoscopy, and was sent to the clinic for assessment instead after all. After the assessment appointment, there was a delay of one week during which Gerald and his wife had to phone the hospital regularly to check on bed availability for Gerald's bronchoscopy. After a week, a bed was found and the bronchoscopy was performed.

3 Gerald was told a week after this by a registrar that he had a 'malignancy' (he did not see the consultant) which *might* be 'treatable' (operable). Several days later, he saw the consultant, who assured him that his cancer was operable and that an operation would be arranged shortly.

4 After another week had gone by with no word from the hospital, Gerald's wife phoned and spoke to the consultant's secretary, who informed them that Gerald was to see a surgeon at a different hospital. The surgeon was on holiday, and there was a long waiting list. The secretary agreed to liaise with the surgeon's secretary to get Gerald in three weeks later for assessment (not for the operation).

5 Gerald's eldest daughter and wife were very upset at the proposed further delay. His daughter rang the secretary back and got the date for assessment moved forward to several days from her call.

6 The appointment card that arrived after this was addressed to the wrong name. On the day of the appointment, no mention of Gerald was found on the appointment list, and he and his wife were told that a new appointment would have to be made.

7 A chance encounter with a receptionist on the way out of the clinic (Gerald explained his situation to her) led her to contact the clinic sister, who unravelled the mistaken identity and found Gerald's missing records which had been sent to the wrong department.

8 Upon their return home, Gerald and his wife found a second-class appointment card waiting with his initial appointment on it (the one that was to have been in three weeks' time).

9 A letter was sent to Gerald with the date of his surgery, but they were instructed to ring the hospital in the intervening time to check on bed availability. On the day Gerald was due to go into hospital, his wife was told to ring from 10.30 am at half-hour intervals throughout the day to see if a bed could be found. After ringing several times she was told there would not be a bed that day. Gerald's daughter (who works in a London hospital) rang various professionals at the hospital where Gerald was to go and was told that there was no guarantee that Gerald's bed would be available the following day either. Her inquiries elicited 'a lecture . . . it was a little, kind of *speech*' from a ward sister about the NHS cutbacks. A bed was found for Gerald.

10 On the day of the surgery (now two and a half months after diagnosis), Gerald's operation was cancelled at the last minute because the surgeon was called away on an emergency (the surgeon came to explain this to Gerald later on that day).

11 Gerald was sent down for surgery the next day, but when he came to he was told that the operation was 'too risky' and had had to be called off (a more thorough bronchoscopy performed on the operating table had revealed inoperability).

12 When Gerald's wife and daughters arrived to see him after the operation, the surgeon took them to a separate room from Gerald and told them that there was nothing he could do for Gerald, saying that the operation was 'too risky'. He also told them that the referring consultant 'had no business' passing Gerald on for surgery and that he would write the man a letter telling him so. Later on, when Gerald began his radiotherapy treatment calendar, the radiotherapy consultant explained the surgeon's reasoning behind his decision not to operate (the tumour was too near the oesophagus).

13 Then, Gerald's initial assessment for radiotherapy at a hospital out-patient combined clinic was called off when it was discovered that his x-rays were missing, and a search in the x-ray department had failed to turn them up. The City A centre radiotherapy consultant whose clinic

> Gerald was attending told him not to worry, and that he would start treatment without the x-rays if need be, after Easter.
>
> 14 Easter had then passed with no word from City A centre. Gerald's wife rang up and the radiotherapy consultant's secretary told her that they were still waiting for Gerald's hospital x-rays, and she suggested they rang the hospital to speak to someone there in the meantime. The person she spoke with at the hospital then insisted that the x-rays had been sent on to City A centre and that there was nothing more they could do. Gerald's wife rang City A centre back and an appointment for Gerald to come in for his set-up for treatment was made immediately.
>
> Gerald, his wife and their daughters said they felt that their combined vigilance had been the only impetus for the surgery treatment calendar in the first place, and that they had been forgotten at the beginning of the illness calendar. By the time Gerald came for his first radiotherapy session, it had been over three months since his diagnosis, during which his wife and daughters had spent considerable time on the telephone trying to arrange his treatment calendar and untangle mix-ups. Gerald's wife said:
>
>> If we hadn't been *ring*ing all this time, what on *earth* would have been done? I just don't understand it, because I would have thought, I mean I've always imagined that, *can*cer, you know that immediately that they'd *do* something. But it certainly hasn't been the case with us. We haven't been able to calm down! It's quite good to be able to talk about it though.

for many people (with the underlying threat of loss of livelihood if the doctor finds 'something serious'), preventing the initiation of the cancer illness calendar.

The ambiguous awareness context pervading the cancer diagnostic course also complicates the experience of becoming diagnosed. This context is constructed by the tendency of professionals to use vague wording and an avoidance of the word 'cancer'. The use of junior staff to relay information and a lack of continuity in whom the patient 'deals with' throughout the course also creates awareness problems. Added to these frequently occurring problems is a pervasive minimization of post-surgical treatment accompanied by a discourse of individualism ('everybody is different') that precludes discussions of such treatment's impact and limitations,[3] and an apparent commitment to keeping the topic of *prognosis* as neutral as possible. Much of this ambiguity is caused by the efforts of clinicians to obscure details that might 'worry' or confuse the patient (McIntosh 1974; Williams 1989; Britten 1991). There appears to be a theoretical commitment among clinicians to 'truth-telling', but an operational assumption that patients don't want to hear or won't understand technical details of illness and treatment.

'Delivery' of the diagnosis

Diagnoses of cancer tend to take place in busy hospital settings, in which there may be problems finding private, quiet space for focused discussion. In the accounts of diagnosis we collected, 'one-off', unambiguous statements of diagnosis (involving initial treatment rationale and prognostic information) delivered in calm and private settings were the exception. Quite often, diagnostic discussions took place in disjointed fashion, on wards and in corridors over a period of days or even weeks as test results were returned and treatability assessed and reassessed. Breast cancer patients seemed to experience the greatest continuity and shortest waiting time from biopsy to diagnostic confirmation and treatment start (though by no means in all cases), whereas lung cancer patients described the most chaotic experiences. Phil, 58, a retired bait farm worker, gives an account of his diagnosis experiences that illustrates several typical contextual features of diagnoses from our sample:

> PH: Well the *first* time that the young one [junior registrar] came to me I was sat in the passage with a couple of fellas and he said, 'I've got some results, do you want to go to your bed?' I says, '*No* it's all right, you can tell me here', you know so, he says, 'Well, you've got a growth on your lung', he just came straight out with it, he didn't beat around the bush *there*, he said, 'We don't foresee any problems, we can remove the lung and you can function on one lung, 'cause the lung has closed itself off, it's not functioning now', and all this you know. Then, he just *went* and uh, it sort of sunk *in*to me and I went back to me bed and I shed a few tears, and one of the staff nurses came up and she says, 'Are you OK?' I said, '*Yeah* I'm OK', she says, 'You're *not*', and she put curtains round and she sat on the bed a few minutes with me you know. I was, I was OK after that like and just, you know when I rung me wife and told me wife like I were a bit upset and that like, but it was after *that* I thought they were ev*a*ding it you know.

Phil is first given diagnostic information by the junior registrar in a corridor (he describes declining the invitation to go somewhere more private). The vague language quoted ('growth') is nevertheless interpreted here as a diagnosis of cancer, and the subsequent minimization of treatment ('we don't foresee any problems, we can remove the lung') gives a clear statement of operability. The abruptness of this interchange ('he just *went* . . . it sort of sunk *in*to me') is offset somewhat by some private time with a sympathetic staff nurse, though the difficult task of breaking the news to Phil's wife is left to him to do alone, over the phone.

Phil described how after this episode he felt left 'in the dark' about his medical status:

PH: They were sort of going round corners you know, like he [junior registrar] came and said after I'd had the scan that surgery was out and then, the next day Dr C came round with a, said some x-rays was missing and he hadn't seen everything and surgery wasn't ruled out and he'd see me later in the day and then, I never even saw him again after that hisself, I just saw his assistant you know and, they were sort of *evad*ing me. In the end, until I pulled them and said, you know, I want to know what's happening, and this is when they told me that I was going to see, they'd made an appointment for me to see Dr D and that. I mean *why* didn't they tell me this right at the beginning? I mean they must have known at the beginning but they didn't tell me. What he [senior registrar at treatment centre] said to me he said, 'Well, you don't really know how to approach people, how they're going to take it', and that.

Phil's subsequent encounters with first the junior registrar and then the consultant are about confusion over the issue of operability (involving wandering x-rays). An assurance of another meeting with the consultant (the senior and 'key' professional) is not honoured ('I never saw him again after that'). Phil describes taking matters into his own hands to force open awareness of his treatment options (operable, or not?) and discovers that he is scheduled to see Dr D, a City A centre radiotherapy consultant. This is apparently interpreted correctly by Phil as a statement of non-operability and therefore of prognostic 'bad news'. Phil's subsequent discussions with the junior registrar assigned to him in hospital, and with Dr D and *his* registrar indicate that the confusion is partly due to their not knowing 'how to approach people, how they're going to *take* it and that'.

Part of the problem in relaying diagnostic information in a decisive and focused manner is that *prognosis* and treatability are always embedded issues, around which there may be considerable medical ambiguity and reassessment by several professionals through the diagnostic process. Gerald, 67, an engineer with lung cancer, also experienced considerable confusion over the issue of operability (which culminated in his being told on the operating table, ready for surgery, that last-minute test results disqualified him for removal of the diseased lung after all). Gerald's diagnosis was embedded in the complex and confusing process of determining operability:

GW: It was one of Dr P's *un*derlings, and he said that the samples had proved malignant.

Wife: He *did* say that several times, along the way, the operation was the best option . . . we had to have another *scan* after that you see . . . it was after the *next* scan that they decided, it was operable.

KCS: Did you understand it *was* cancer when they said malignancy?

GW: *Oh* yes, heh heh, no question about *that*, we knew what that was.

Wife: He *did* say, the registrar, that it's a form of lung cancer that's *treat*able, because that's the only *time*, I think anybody has said lung *can*cer actually.

Here an initially vague statement ('the samples had proved malignant') delivered by 'one of Dr P's underlings' is followed by the suggestion that an operation is an option for Gerald, and this is apparently confirmed by a subsequent CT scan. Gerald's wife recalls one registrar's use of the word 'cancer' as unique. In fact, Gerald's case was plagued with every small disaster that can befall a patient en route to diagnosis and treatment for cancer (see the case summary in Box 3.1).

When surgery was finally ruled out (literally at the last minute), Gerald's waiting family are summoned to the hospital to hear the bad news:

Wife: We didn't find him (the surgeon) so, Mr M =

GW: = Not initially =

Wife: = friendly, no we didn't find him so when we came *down*, course *we* got a shock. Me two daughters came up from London, and so we'd been filling the day, and we'd just walked in and got this phone call from the hospital and, I mean she said to me, 'Well, Mr M hasn't proceeded with the operation, have you got someone *there* with you?' Well that, *terr*ified me straight away you know, I mean me daughters are here. She says, 'Well he'd like to see you.' So we went, we went down, the three of us and he was still talking to you, Gerald, when we got there, and heh! He, he walked over . . . he walked [gets up and demonstrates] towards us like *that*, and just turned and walked into the room and we followed like, little *lambs* you know I mean if he'd just sort of, put his hand on, our shoulder or, or said come now, let's go sit with you . . . but he *nev*er spoke, he just, turned on his heel and walked in and we followed like =

GW: = Sheep to the slaughter.

Gerald and his wife went on to describe the surgeon's apparent disgust over the referring consultant's poor assessment of Gerald's situation, and his feelings of having been given the difficult job of explaining the mistake to Gerald and his family:

Wife: Somewhere along the line I, I think that Mr M was, *I* got the impression that he was a bit cross, *with* Dr P [referring consultant], with *paint*ing the picture so

GW: Rosy

Wife: So glowing, 'cause he said to *us* he said, 'Well I'm not going to do it. I mean,' he says, 'it's all right for the GPs you know and the specialists along the way, but you see it stops *here*,' and he says, 'I'm the one who gets left with you know, having to *tell* people that, if this doesn't work out . . .' In fact I *think* he wrote to Dr P. It was a borderline one. I always remember when he *said* that it was operable . . . I mean we were elated really, sounds a funny thing but, I mean we thought, might be it could be *cured*.

Gerald and his wife both described much improved communication with the surgeon after this initial difficult encounter, citing as crucial the lengthy amounts of time he spent talking to them in subsequent meetings.

Because of the medical ambiguity that typically attends early assessments of prognosis and treatment options, diagnostic experiences can involve several professionals, many tests, different hospital departments (and occasionally different institutions), exploratory surgery, and time spent waiting for results. In this often complex context, liaison between professionals and patients and with their family members is considerably compromised. Bronwyn, 58, a housewife with a chortoid (eye) tumour, and her husband reported never receiving a statement of diagnosis of *cancer*, in the flurry of activity following her sudden experience of eye pain and subsequent removal of the eye:

Husband: Well, initially it's all *vague*. I would have thought that Mr N [surgeon] would have had a word to tell me what it *was*, even if he didn't have a word with Bronwyn, but he *didn't* . . . what we wanted to know was, was it malignant or was it a benign tumour and *that* we couldn't find out . . . it was only when we saw Dr D [radiotherapy consultant] at [City A] that he said that she was having radium treatment for . . . and I banged this to cancer and then realised that it *was* malignant.

KCS: Sometimes it's difficult because you don't know what to ask?

BG: After the person's gone you think *ooh* I should have asked *this* you know . . .

Husband: And all the people that *I* could ask when I've visited the hospital in visiting hours is the ward staff, and they just didn't know, or, they pretended they didn't know. Obviously, I couldn't get information off the telephone and I asked the staff nurse who was a young fella, *he* was very good as well, and *he* couldn't tell me, and I said would you ask Mr N a specific question for me, so that you can answer it for me when I visit this afternoon? Anyway when I got there there was no message 'cause this is what I wanted to know – was it malignant or benign, and I *just* could not get to know.

In the absence of clear discussions about or statements of diagnosis, patients look to aspects of the diagnostic process and the proposed treatment calendar for confirmation that they have *cancer*. Adam, 58, a retired textile worker with lung cancer, describes first deducing the nature of his illness from the extent of the surgery initially suggested by the consultant, prior to diagnostic confirmation by the surgeon following bronchoscopy:

AL: Mr W referred me to hospital to, a Mr M [surgeon], who I saw within about 10 days, he was on holiday at the time, and that was the first time I *knew*, when I saw Mr M on that day that it was malignant, because I came out of the hospital before the result had come *back*. Although, I *knew* in me own *mind* that, from what Dr W had said, you know like, it *would* be malignant, because he was on about me lung coming out, and I was strong enough to take it and this, that and the other. So *you* know, it was, more or less in me own mind that it *was* that. I only got to know, didn't we [to wife], when we saw Mr M.

The statement of diagnosis recounted by Adam from this surgeon was that the 'suspicions' of the referring consultant 'had been confirmed', but no mention of the word 'cancer'.

In many cases there is apparently no confirmation of a diagnosis of cancer. Rather, awareness dawns as a result of events in the early illness calendar, professionals' manner, types of treatment discussed, and details of the treatment calendar. Some of these are described by Jim, 63, a saw operator who had been receiving laser treatment for what was initially said to be a urinary tract wart:

KCS: When you heard the, the bit about the 'growth', that was sort of, when you twigged that =

JW: = No that was when I saw Mr I [surgeon] look uneasy. And then when I got this letter from Mr I saying that, come back and then let's do this and that and he'd decided I needed more, treatment in the form of radio*therapy*, and he had been in touch with his colleague Dr D [radiotherapy consultant] and in due course I would *hear* from Dr D, and in fact I'd already *heard* from him . . . well, they got crossed up a little bit *some*where. As I say I had an appointment to go to *see* Dr D [at City A Treatment Centre] before I got the letter from Mr I to put me in touch with him. I had to visit me *own* GP to, ask him what it was *about*, and *he* couldn't tell – it was to tell me when I could come *in* [for radiotherapy] ... And that was when I obviously *knew* that I'd got, it was something a little bit more serious than a *wart*.

It was not unusual for patients or their GPs to receive letters from the City A centre about starting radiotherapy treatment *before* they had been told they had cancer.

In several cases, it appeared that a diagnosis of cancer had not so much been *given*, as assumed by the various professionals involved (indeed, three patients had been monitored and treated for cancer for one to two years before apparently finding out that their illnesses *were* cancer); relaying a diagnosis was sometimes no one person's 'job' in particular. By Jim's account, in early discussions with the hospital consultant, the technically explicit object of the x-ray was kept obscure by the consultant's avoidance of the word 'cancer':

JW: *May*be you're just supposed to *guess*. I mean they just point something out on an x-ray and say *that*'s the problem, that growth has got to come out and you're supposed to guess what it *is*.

KCS: So you feel as though you could have been =

JW: = Well I mean if he'd said, that is cancer it's got to come out, then you know where you are.

Patients often have to deal with confusing and contradictory information even in cases where they are expressly told they have cancer. Some descriptions of patients' encounters with consultants and surgeons seemed to suggest that a certain 'staging' of awareness was favoured by these professionals, rather than clear statements about diagnosis and prognosis (or acknowledgement of test result ambiguity). Rachael, 41, a supply teacher, was initially told by her surgeon of the treatment options available *if* her breast lump was found to be malignant, including mastectomy. He then sent a letter to her GP describing the lump as 'suspicious', information she received only while consulting the GP for one of her children:

RS: Well, I did have to see my doctor in between time [between biopsy and surgery] with one of the children and *he* said that he'd had a letter from Mr H saying that it was suspicious which, made me think a little bit more a*bout* it, oh well, maybe it's not just harmless. So there was a lot ... you know I was suspicious, but *then*, the morning of the operation [lumpectomy] Mr H *did* come round and he did say it was be*nign*, or the sample they'd taken was benign, and I think you know I be-*liev*ed that, 'cause I'd believed all along it was going to be nothing. So I think it was more of a *shock*, afterwards.

KCS: Afterwards, what happened? Do you remember what he said?

> RS: Well *no*, I mean I haven't seen Mr H since. His registrar I think
> it was. He was one of four doctors that used to come round,
> I think he was the one in *charge*. Well the *first* indication that
> I had was, I felt that I'd been under the anaesthetic for a long
> time, much longer than I should have been . . . none of the nurses
> had said anything and that, and I think I phoned my husband
> up to say good morning to the kids, and he said that he'd seen
> the nurse and *she* said that I was probably going to be in *long*er
> than we'd expected . . . and then, when the doctor came round,
> on his rounds he said that you know it was, a tumour, a lump,
> a lump maybe. I don't think cancer was actually mentioned.

Here, Rachael describes a confusing and contradictory process, in which
information is hard to come by, particularly from the central treatment
professional.

Helen, 63, a housewife, went to hospital to have a second mammogram
after a routine visit had turned up a tiny lump in her breast. She describes
finding the surgeon's statement of a worst case scenario and subsequent
choice of a more minor lumpectomy comforting:

> HB: While I was *there*, and they were thinking about this, Mr H
> came to see me, and didn't say, what it *was*, but he didn't say it
> *was*n't, and he explained what it *might* be and what they *might*
> do, including a complete mastectomy, and in the same *breath*,
> before I'd a chance to draw breath meself he says but we would
> do an implant. You know I didn't have a chance to think *ooh
> gosh* what will they do? I'm very thankful for that, he's very
> good. Then, later on in the evening he came up and my husband
> was there, and uh, he's done some work on my husband, he
> recognized him, so of course, quite a family reunion in a way,
> heh! He'd *got* the result and he confirmed that it was cancer, and
> he said that there's *no* question of a mastectomy though because
> he knew how much there *was*.

Helen and her husband already had a relationship with the surgeon and
this perhaps facilitated a more relaxed discussion. Ellie, 64, a retired catering
assistant, and her husband describe their meeting with this same surgeon
and a similar provision of a 'worst case scenario':

> Husband: Cancer was never mentioned.
> ER: They took the stitches out, then Mr H said, 'Will you come
>   into this office', and the, sister went with us. And then, he
>   looked over his glasses like this, heh! and said, I don't
>   know what he said, but we all got the idea, we all knew,
>   but I can't really tell you what he said.
> Husband: *No* I was waiting for him *using* the word ['cancer'] and he
>   *nev*er, he said, whatever it *was*, they found something, in

the *cent*re, which was quite a thin head, and then this long *pause* wasn't there? [inhales loudly] you see, *noth*ing, now do *I* shout up or, or what? So, everybody's waiting for one another to say something, and he said to her, he never mentioned the word, he said, 'So, there is an option, and I'm pretty confident that I've taken everything away, there's nothing left but' =

ER: = *But*

Husband: 'Just to make *sure*, that I got it all . . . you *do* know what a "belt and braces job" is don't you?'

ER: The treatment that I've had is an in*sur*ance that there's nothing left, or, we can do a mastectomy – *well* I nearly, I just couldn't be*lieve* that, I said well, how can you compare the two *things*? I mean if he'd, said that he'd re*moved* the lump and as far as he was concerned, it was *clear*, I mean there was su— it was such an early stage and *yet* he's mentioning having a mas*tec*tomy . . . oh it seems such a drastic thing to *do*.

While the word 'cancer' is not recalled by Ellie and her husband, other technical details of the visit are (in fact, patients and their spouses tended to use the appropriate medical terminology when discussing diagnosis and treatment quite accurately). In the excerpt, the surgeon is described as juxtaposing the lumpectomy and radiotherapy treatment (Ellie had had a lumpectomy and was about to begin radiotherapy at the time of the interview) with mastectomy as equivalent treatment 'options'. The implied equation of the two forms of treatment, amid assurances that the original lumpectomy was successful, is described by Ellie as absurd: why would she choose mastectomy if the lumpectomy had 'got it all'?

Ellie's characterization of radiotherapy as 'an in*sur*ance that there's nothing left' follows the way in which many treatment professionals characterize post-surgical treatment. How can a treatment that is mere 'insurance' be a logical alternative to the more 'drastic' mastectomy? The issue of treatment 'choice' only ever arose in the interview accounts of breast cancer patients, who described 'options' presented as '*faits accompli*' by their surgeons. Choice in the diagnostic context remains so obscure as to be almost a non-issue, like prognosis, rarely discussed explicitly. The patient is likely to receive the treatment mode(s) espoused by the individual clinician (and treatment centre) rather than make an informed choice from an array of presented choices. Here Gail, 36, a housewife, describes her 'choice' of lumpectomy for her breast cancer:

KCS: Do you think you've had information, to be able to make decisions, or to feel like you've been involved in the decision-making process?

GR: Uhmm, well I suppose I was given a choice, I mean I was given a choice by Dr P to have a, radiotherapy or have a mastectomy. But I'd also said, I said, 'But you've taken all the, cancer out presumably', and he said, 'Yes, this is just to be on the safe side, just in case.' So I said, 'Oh there's not much point in a mastectomy really is there!' I mean, if that's a choice, I suppose.

Describing treatment in such cosy terms as 'precaution' and 'like an insurance policy', while temporarily protecting patients from worry, was in direct contrast with the reality of the exigencies of treatment, as Martha, 48, a factory worker with floor-of-mouth cancer, describes:

MS: I thought it were only going to be a small operation, you know. I think he misled me a little bit did Mr B [surgeon] but it happens well he did. He said, we're just going to *cut* there love, and we're going to take a little *piece* out of here a little piece out of your arm, put it back of your throat, and, just nick down here. I thought *ah* that's not that bad. And then I wakened up in there *I* got the devil of a shock.

Martha came close to dying in the intensive care unit following the operation. She expressed gratitude and admiration for the surgeon's efforts to remove the cancer and reconstruct her face, and for his personal attention following the operation. Such operations are the product of greatly improved surgical techniques and expertise that significantly improve the chances of survival from a particularly voracious form of maxillofacial cancer. However, it is questionable whether a paternalistic minimization of such treatment is helpful to the patient.

Diagnosis is often part of a context of early treatment that involves significant suffering and loss. The tasks of both revealing and hearing diagnostic information are complicated when, in addition to the cancer diagnosis itself, the patient must face the loss of a body part and/or permanent loss of function. Much has been noted about the trauma of losing a breast to mastectomy (playing a part in the current emphasis on lumpectomy and radiotherapy instead for these patients), yet there are many other cancers the treatment of which involves even more ravaging losses. Lung cancer patients can face loss of a lung with the attendant reduction in function. Maxillofacial cancer patients can deal with great disfigurement and loss of function in seeing, eating, speaking, tasting and breathing. Patients with floor-of-mouth cancer have all their teeth extracted before undergoing extensive facial surgery, involving large skin grafts taken from their arms. Patients with cancer of the larynx often face removal of the larynx if radiotherapy is unsuccessful in eradicating the cancer. A woman from our sample lost her eye to a chortoid tumour and had to be fitted with a prosthesis. The shock of extensive surgery involving physical loss (disfiguring, function-reducing and permanent) is a factor in the diagnostic context that complicates handling of the diagnosis itself by patients, their families and professionals, as more is being responded to than the *fact* of the cancer (loss of 'health', and potential loss of life) alone.

Diagnosis as a definitional problem for the diagnosed

The definitional tasks of patients and family members, once a diagnosis of cancer is intuited or understood, involve working out the significance of treatment calendars, including the results of tests and examinations, in relation to a 'seriousness context', or an idea of prognosis. Determining the seriousness of one's illness is a difficult task for many patients, because of how very *well* they may feel physically. Low-level symptoms, improved detection technology and the effectiveness of early treatment all mean that the person newly diagnosed for cancer may feel no different from usual. In addition to establishing a seriousness context, the newly diagnosed person must work out a context within which illness calendar experience (which has largely supplanted the ordinary rhythms of living) and the illness itself – issues of 'symptoms' and cause – can be seen as meaningful, rational and *liveable*. Both these tasks involve the activity (becoming, often, a strategy) of dimensionalizing: comparing and contrasting with the experience of others in the treatment setting and the community, and assessing the information gained from both contexts. Through the social process of dimensionalizing, a social context within which to locate personal experience is developed. Dimensionalizing and building a context necessarily involve clarifying ambiguity and striving for more open awareness.

Developing a context of 'seriousness'

Melissa, 49, a housekeeper at a university student residence, describes community disclosure of cancer in response to news of her breast lumpectomy. Her account is typical of many patients', of suddenly discovering an experience with cancer in their neighbourhoods they had not heard of before:

> *MG:* . . . Whilst I was in the [dentist's] chair he says to me my *wife's* just had that operation. I said good *hell* you never, he said *yes*, 18 months ago he said she's doing *fine*. When I came *out* of the dentist, his wife had even popped – they live, not far – she even popped over to introduce herself, which I thought was *very* kind really . . . there's a lady up the road actually, and it was funny because I didn't know *she'd* had it, but as I was walking back from the paper shop one Sunday morning she just stopped me

and asked, how's Fred? [husband], and you know I sort of spoke to her and she said *oh* well I just had my breast off for cancer, and so I said good *grief*, so, you look at people like *that*. I mean, a couple of them tend to be older than what *I* am, so I sort of think to myself, well, if people like *that* can have it and get over it . . .

. . . because you know until you sort of, meet up with people like that, *you* just don't think about it in ordinary everyday life . . . and yet whilst I was *in* there [hospital], I saw on a scale you just cannot *believe*, what really goes on. *You* know, I mean *every*body but *every*body is just run off their *feet*, and I mean seeing them going up and down to that operating theatre, well it's just like looking at them on the *motor*way, going up and down on them trolleys. You just don't think about that sort of thing, that's going on *in* there.

These disclosures can provide Melissa with the beginnings of a context within which she can locate herself, one quite different from the 'ordinary everyday life' outside the hospital, prediagnosis. This context will be necessary increasingly, as Melissa gives voice here to her unwillingness to directly question her doctors or to 'know too much':

MG: I've seen Mr H [surgeon] but, not to ask anything about the operation. In all fairness, I'm one of these people that, I leave it in *their* hands, I don't really like to ask a lot of questions because, if there's anything I don't really want to know I'd rather they didn't *tell* me, if you know what I mean. Really, I think that's being a silly way to look at it, but, having said that, I'm a terrible worrier, I worry *aw*ful.

Melissa described her code as, 'never trouble trouble until trouble troubles you'. A similar approach to the issue of 'knowing too much' (and risking having to hear a poor prognosis) is described by May, 53, a pub caterer with floor-of-mouth cancer:

MG: And so, but my husband heard these two younger doctors, I don't know who they are, they looked too old to be *stu*dents, but they didn't look as im*por*tant as *oth*ers you know. And, he heard one say t'other what, what they'd *done* with me. But he also says it, has gone very very deep and that B [surgeon] – cause it were deeper than he'd thought, he'd had to go very deep to get it – I mean, there must have been summat said along the *way*, or a note mustn't there, for 'em to *know*?

KCS: But is that something you weren't aware of?

MG: Well no and all, I *was*n't really, no – I don't like to get B, I'm not getting him into bother am I? Cause there were a few things, but there again as I say it could be my own fault, cause I didn't *ask* I didn't ad*dress* you know.

KCS: Well, yeah, it can be difficult to know what to ask.

MG: *Oh*, I knew what questions to ask, I didn't want to hear the answers to 'em. Well, *yeah* it could be difficult because, I mean *I* didn't know about, having to have your *veins* out, and, I wouldn't have *thought* of uh, asking that you know, or anything like that.

May here describes finding out about a more severe situation than her initial discussions with the surgeon had intimated, and speculates about how the 'younger doctors' came to know it. She had had to have a section of flesh including a working vein cut from her arm and attached to her face to cover the hole left by the tumour excision. While many of the details of the complicated surgery had eluded her, she describes her basic reluctance to question the surgeon as not wanting to hear the answers to her questions. Many patients described their reluctance to know more while simultaneously exploring in interview their fears, guesses, and interpretations of the meaning of the developing treatment calendar: 'How ill am I?'.

Interpreting significance and filling in blanks

Part of the problem for patients and their families in answering this question is the social situation of diagnosis and post-operative recovery. The lack of private spaces and time for discussions with key professionals is a feature of this situation, as well as the apparent avoidance of intimacy by these professionals, as described in patient accounts. Here Meg, a 50 year-old housewife with breast cancer describes her surgeon's manner on ward rounds:

MT: Everybody says how nice [the surgeon] is and, all this. Yes, he's all right, he jokes but, I think, how can I say it? he's not direct at you. He always brings his gang with him, you know what I mean, his housemen and all the rest. He'll just say, say *about* it, but *joke* and then, up and go, you know what I mean?

Information that *is* directly asked for is often hard to interpret in the absence of a context to make sense of details. While most patients are ultimately aware, as the diagnostic process proceeds, of their *diagnosis*, they are frequently *un*aware of the significance of diagnostic information. Such information as how extensive the disease is, precisely where the involvement is, whether there is any evidence of spread, what the significance of having positive nodes is and how many all has prognostic significance.

Ellie, 64, a retired catering assistant, describes trying to determine the size of her breast tumour:

> ER: I wish I could keep quiet and wait for them to tell me things, but I *don't*. I said, how big was it? Was it like a pea? I mean I don't know what's big or little *really*. And he said yes. So I mean, I don't know whether that's big or little, I don't know anything about, anything *else* you see.

In the absence of a context for interpretation, everything professionals say becomes potentially significant. Adam, 58, a retired textile worker with lung cancer, and his wife describe trying to interpret a turn of phrase used often by professionals during examinations:

> Wife: This *last* time when [the radiotherapy consultant's] assistant examined him, *she* said the same, 'oh good, very good'. So, [Adam] did say but *is* it *good* because we'd hear them say it *so* often you know. *I* don't know really what her answer was, do you? [to Adam].
>
> AL: She just says 'oh yeah, very good', so what was very good I don't *know*.

Patients' accounts suggest a reluctance to press professionals for more information when their questions are answered vaguely. Those that described persisting after initial brush-offs sometimes found help, but usually from lower-status professionals, like nurses and radiographers at the treatment centre. Here Chris, 49, an electrician with cancer of the larynx, describes a contrast between his talks with the surgeon and senior registrar at the hospital, and those with the treatment centre's 'maskman' (the technician responsible for making treatment masks for head and neck cancer patients) and other staff at the radiotherapy simulator machine.:

> CB: This is [the surgeon's] ass*i*stant, *oh* he says, well it's only a *small* one and I said well, what's a *small* one? I says is it bigger than a walnut, or what? He says *oh* you've no need to worry, he said, there's people worse off than *you*. I wouldn't think that's the right attitude from a physician, a bedside manner like *that*, with things like, with *cancer* . . .

Later on, he had spoken with the surgeon himself:

> CB: Well, as far as I know, I think they cut part of the tumour off. When I *asked* him why he didn't cut it *all* off – it seemed *strange* to me – he says, oh well, at [treatment centre] they need something to *aim* at. That seemed a bit strange to me, but then I don't know the technical details . . . he just seemed to be by-passing through the ward, you know *how* are things going, so-and-so, well you'll be alright now and then they go on to the *next* bed

you know. I would have liked to have known how I was cut up and not 'it's not a very big lump and, people worse off than you'. I mean if I was doing work for somebody now in *my* profession, then I'd think they're entitled to know as much as I *think* they can take in and understand.

Chris described having a lot of questions when he came to the centre to have his mask made prior to starting radiotherapy. The technicians he spoke with were responsible for fitting patients with masks to wear during treatment, and had apparently explained the various ways radiation was used to treat tumours like his:

CB: They explained what they do. They said we'll draw you a little map, and, you know, cause I wondered, if you look at your vocal chords, you can see them go like that [shows v-shape of vocal chords]. And he explained, how they *treat* it. What they took today [images from a treatment simulator machine] was just a, what they do to check their accuracy you see, they practice it, and he explained that . . . as I say, I didn't even know why it was called *cancer* until they said it's – it appears to be, the actual cell formation looks like a little crawling crab, so I learnt something else as well from them.

It was intimated in accounts that the underlying threat of a poor prognosis shaped patients' quest for greater awareness of the situation. Gaps or changes in the treatment calendar were frequently interpreted as indications of 'seriousness' (disease spread, reduced treatability), as Phil describes here:

PH: I *think* [the cancer] is just outside the lung because at first they were going to remove it and then they said that they couldn't so it must be just outside. When they first did the tests and found the growth in the lung, they said you know doing further tests and if there's nothing else then we remove the lung, there's no problem. Well there *must* be because, they decided they couldn't *remove* it, so . . .

The treatment calendar is deeply significant within an ambiguous awareness context, as it serves as the main source of information allowing the patient to locate herself within a 'seriousness' context. A frequently-voiced concern of patients undergoing radical radiotherapy was why their courses were so long in relation to those having only several days' treatment. Their interpretation of this difference focused on their being 'more ill' than those treated less, whereas in fact the reverse was usually the case.

The process of filling in blanks and interpreting significance was largely a *covert* one. The rationale for ordering x-rays and scans was rarely provided, and there were no clear mechanisms for patients and family members to find out the results. Results were often sent from one institution to another, or between units within the hospital, and there seemed little protocol for relaying them to the patient. Nina, 61, a housewife with breast cancer, describes her persistence in finding out results of tests on her removed lymph glands:

> NS: I did ask [the surgeon] were there any results through. He was abrupt. Uh *no* no there isn't. He didn't explain that it would be so *long*, that I wouldn't hear until I got to [City A Centre]. We were hoping our doctor would get a letter and *he* would tell me. But we inquired but he *had*n't got a letter, we inquired before we left the hospital but he hadn't heard. They didn't *say*, but I guessed I had to wait until I got to [City A], and as time went on, you knew well *that* will be it, it *would* be [City A].

Issues involving 'seriousness' and prognosis are, of course, 'life and death' issues for the patient, whereas they are important technical issues for the clinician. Interpreting significance and filling in blanks are central tasks for patients to face in locating themselves in a meaningful context within the illness calendar. Professionals are engaged in finding out information about prognosis in preparation for the treatment trajectory, but this activity goes on 'above the patient's head' so to speak, and is largely inaccessible to him.

Establishing cause and re-interpreting 'symptoms'

Context-building among patients was heard to involve the discussion of possible causal factors and the re-evaluation of physical instability experienced prior to learning the diagnosis. In this way, instability *became* symptomatic of the cancer. This re-working of experience in light of others' definitions is a central feature of the social construction of illness (Seiden Miller 1978). In this way, patients' accounts of 'symptoms' and cause strove to depict cancer as *accountable*, rather than a chaotic happening that had suddenly simply occurred. While these two definitional tasks were given a prominent place in interviews by the patients, little support for them was reported as coming from 'key' treatment professionals (those most central to the planning of the treatment calendar). Certain lower-status professionals we have called 'helpers in the trajectory' were described as helpful in the definitional work of patients, and more will be said about them in Chapters 4 and 5.

Treatment professionals seemed to have dismissed the issue of cause as inconsequential, especially in light of a poor prognosis for many cancers, and given the *fact* of the cancer and the work needed to be done in treating it. Little is understood about causal processes and factors in the majority of cancers. Much is made in both the health promotion literature and the popular press of 'lifestyle' as a cause of serious illness, especially 'habits' like smoking, drinking, and eating poorly. Alternative sources of cause, like poor working conditions, pollution and poverty (and the ways in which these intersect with those of 'lifestyle') are more politically sensitive and more rarely discussed. Also, as in the case of unpredictable outcomes of treatment and the unpredictable disease course, professionals are reluctant to speculate on a subject about which little is known (McIntosh 1974; Williams 1989).

There are diverse reasons for patients' apparent interest in the issue of cause. Understanding causal factors is often important in making life changes once cancer is diagnosed, like stopping smoking (although there is still a lack of organised medical support for patients making these changes). Establishing some understanding of cause was also essential in placing the cancer in the context of a long period of physical suffering (like that brought on by a difficult menopause prior to diagnosis of breast cancer, for example), or in relation to a stressful life event (like losing a spouse). Attempts at establishing cause had to do in some way with answering the question, 'Why *me* and not somebody else *like* me?'.

Speculation about cause was a way of exploring the unknown as well as seeing the cancer as a rational event – an event with an understandable cause. Many people voiced the concern that cause was important because of their place in their family's illness history ('Will my children become ill too?') or as 'the one who had cancer' if they had been the only one. The issue of cause has implications for personal identity, and for how the rest of the family deals with the diagnosis. Here Betty, 44, a retired WREN, voices concerns about the cause of her breast cancer:

BG: Yes, I want to know what causes it. So now, that's the next step. I've got my theories. Menopausal. I know I've been through the menopause, now I started early. So I've been going on 5 years. Well, it's a big shake-up to your body. And why have I got it and my mother hasn't? I'm the only one in the family, even going back.

Working out cause may be subtly bound up with the issue of what *might* have happened if one 'hadn't found out' about the cancer. Helen, 63, a housewife whose breast cancer was asymptomatic and diagnosed through mammography said that she felt she had 'blotted the copybook' for her family as the only one known to have had cancer. Here she describes confusion about the development of cancer in her breast:

HB: So goodness knows when I'd have found mine because it was so small. The *frightening* thing about it was that it *was* so small and yet it – I said to [the surgeon] what came *first* you know, was it a *lump* that went that way, or what. He said well, it probably started, both started together. So the cancer cells must have got in there, and made the lump, which is very frightening, and I don't like it very much.

Helen describes being left with the disturbing idea that her breast had been invaded from outside by the cancer. These types of accounts suggested that many patients (with varying prognoses) saw their diagnosis as a fortuitous accident without which they would have been in great danger. The 'lucky' diagnosis was seen as having saved them from a hostile future (Silverman and Perakyla 1990) in which they would have been at much greater risk through ignorance of the cancer.

Establishing cause is sometimes linked to a struggle for resources for patients and families, in cases where the cancer has a possible connection to environmental factors. In our sample, Gary, 60, had been a plumber for two institutions and had contracted mesothelioma (asbestos cancer) through working with asbestos lagging, unprotected, over a period of twenty years. The cause of Gary's cancer was indisputable, but resolving his compensation case was hung up on the legal problem of which institution to find at fault, and he was likely to die before a solution was found. Adam, 58, diagnosed with lung cancer, had worked in the textile industry in a village near City A. Six of his friends and co-workers, all of retirement age and living in that same village had been diagnosed with cancers of the head and neck, and lung, and a seventh had died from lung cancer. In cases such as these, establishing cause becomes a social issue, one involving the allocation of resources, and one with wider social implications.

Many patients described how the absence of pain and the innocuous nature of their physical instability (and the often non-linear nature of their diagnostic process) caused confusion as to what had or had not been a 'symptom' of the cancer. Adam, who had angina, had had what his GP thought was a viral flu which had made him nauseated, and produced weight loss, which he assumed to be from not eating. Here, he and his wife describe being confused by the senior registrar's response to their questions about his cancer 'symptoms':

> Wife: I said what are the symptoms, she said well he *had* the symptoms, I thought she was a bit, that's the only time I thought anybody was a bit *sharp*. She said well, he *had* the symptoms, he's got to have them for them to have sent him to hospital. I said, well *no*, the doctor sent him to the hospital because of his *heart* complaint, and then at the check-up he was taken for a *virus*...

Concern over interpretation of 'symptoms' is also related to the fear that the cancer may have spread. Alice, 58, a business owner and manager who had described experiencing problems with her breasts for a two-year period before finally being diagnosed with cancer, asked her radiotherapy consultant about whether her instability could have been related to the cancer:

> AW: He assures me he said, *he* doesn't think it's a symptom. But after all, it's ended up being cancer, because the *skin* was funny. It wasn't wrinkled but almost wrinkled, sort of light and dark shading. And when I was sat in the bath and sat the other way it wasn't on the other side, do you know what I mean? Cause Dr D [consultant] said wasn't it on the other side? Then there was a dimple, when I lifted the flesh and somebody said to me, it attaches itself to the skin, now Dr D poo-pooed *that* . . . [Alice describes her 2 years of instability pre-menopause] and I felt like this for a long *time* and *that's* what eventually made me go see the doctor. And I've had headaches, which I never suffered from before – this is what makes me wonder if it's gone further.

Here, Alice speculates about how she feels – is it menopause or metastasized cancer? Her two years of unsettling physical instability and a brother terminally ill with an inoperable brain tumour make her concern understandable. Interestingly, all the breast irregularities she describes are textbook symptoms of malignancy in the breast, yet are apparently discounted by the clinician when she raises these with him. In a climate of ambiguous awareness, in which the issue of prognosis is neutralized or non-existent in consultations, suspicion and fear about spread may lead a worried patient to interpret many 'symptoms' as signs of advanced disease.

In our studies, the voiced interest of patients and their families to discuss the issues of cause and symptoms appeared to have gone largely unheeded in the busy diagnostic and treatment settings of their early illness calendars. There is a pervasive sense in which issues of ætiology are considered the exclusive province of medical *science*, and not specifically relevant to day-to-day medical *practice* in the treatment of cancer. Also, there is a pragmatic emphasis in the medical setting (with its limited resources for which there is endless competition and demand) on 'getting on with' the immediate tasks at hand: treating an existing and life-threatening condition. This pragmatism however, dis-allows patients' concerns over the ambiguous nature of their illnesses. In this sense, clinical medicine does *not* concern itself with the causes of chronic illnesses, rather only with their effects (cause is seen as an academic issue – not a major concern for the clinical treatment situation). This one-dimensionality, although arising out of inherent limitations of medical knowledge and resources, does the patient an injustice, because within such a context, much that is of central importance to the patient is omitted from the clinical gaze. Discussions about cause have real uses and implications for patients, even if the determination of causes is ultimately ambiguous or impossible, and even if 'nothing can be done' about them.

Summary

In light of the basic complexity of the cancer diagnosis process, especially as regards the ambiguous awareness context pervading it, the point emerges that diagnoses (including attendant prognostic and treatment rationale information) are not so much *given* by clinicians to patients, as they are *revealed* (usually only partially) by clinicians and interpreted by patients. This distinction is important; clinicians choose how to relay details of the diagnosis and *which* details to expose to the patient's awareness, which to leave out. There is no unitary entity called a 'diagnosis' – just a process, often untidy or difficult, reported upon by clinicians to patients, in which the most pressing issue is how best to maximize the patient's chances for survival, or, in other words, prognosis. There are many issues related to this central one of prognosis that we found to have been largely left unvoiced in the diagnostic and early treatment experiences of patients, including detailed discussions of the effects of treatments and the permanent changes they bring to the lives of patients and families, extensiveness of disease and tissue involvement, explanations of tests and procedures and their interpretation, details of post-treatment follow-up, and treatment options and their comparative benefits and drawbacks.

The diagnostic and early treatment planning process is constructed around managing awareness of prognosis. This management of awareness may include obscuring awareness of the *diagnosis* itself, but it will certainly involve limiting the awareness of the *meaning* of procedures and information as this relates to prognosis. Both the illness *and* the early illness calendar, as a new social situation, present the patient and family with many tasks of interpretation. Illness calendar agents play a central role in the construction of awareness, both aiding and blocking patients' efforts towards interpretation and definition. Another block to awareness is the pragmatic emphasis of the medical setting, in which issues or concerns from 'outside' the immediate medical agenda are discounted. Such concerns, it is argued here and in the following pages, have a direct bearing on how patients and families manage and experience the treatment calendar, and on the impact of the treatment calendar on their personal calendars. Another way of saying this is that such concerns have direct relevance for 'quality of life' of patients and families.

Notes

1 Knudtson and Suzuki (1992: 143), in their discussion of 'Western' vs. indigenous peoples' conceptions of time, point out that in the West, the conventional concept of time is '. . . linear, sequential, and unidirectional, like an arrow, speeding away from the taut bowstring that launched it toward its unseen target, never to

retrace its trajectory'. In this context, the pervasiveness of the calendar in daily life is easy to understand: its abstraction permits us the feeling that we have control of the relentless forward movement of the endlessly fleeing arrow. In contrast, the West's native peoples have traditionally seen time as cyclical, following the rhythms of nature. Through their marking of these circular phases and fluctuations through ritual,

> ... the primeval cycles of nature – and circular time itself – are symbolically renewed and rendered 'eternally present' – in essence, timeless. Far from being reduced to abstractions, they are personally and collectively *experienced* as living ecological and spiritual cycles of time.
>
> (Knudtson and Suzuki 1992: 144)

2 The reader may here be reminded of the work of Nerenz and Levanthal (1983) on cognitive representations of illness. They describe such representations as composed of four main constructions, the *identity* of an illness (its name and symptoms), and beliefs about its *causes*, *duration* and *consequences* for personal life.

3 While patients assume, unless expressly told otherwise (and such frankness is scarce in the early treatment calendar) that their treatment calendars will be 'radical' or aimed at 'cure', and that this goal informs clinicians' judgements of appropriate treatments and calendars, this may not be the case. For example, radiotherapy is not found greatly to influence overall survival in women with breast cancer, because it does not limit the likelihood of metastatic disease; rather, it is effective in preventing local recurrence of the tumour in the breast (Horwich and Duchesne 1988). One does not die from a breast tumour, but from the effects of metastatic disease. This raises the question of why extensive radiotherapy (3–5 weeks) is routinely given following lumpectomy (the two seem to be presented as a 'package' in treatment discussions). Local recurrence is thought by clinicians to be sufficiently disturbing that preventing it is seen as an important treatment goal. However, the point emerges that women should perhaps be given clearer information as to the limitations of radiotherapy's effect on prognosis.

4 Getting started: preparing for life in the treatment calendar

In the previous chapter we focused on the early illness calendar dominated by the process of coming to a diagnosis. Surgery and assessments of treatability complicate the patients' coming to terms with the diagnosis. As the illness calendar progresses beyond the point of diagnosis, preparations for post-surgical treatment must be made. This chapter focuses on the preparations for lengthy radiotherapy and chemotherapy treatment that must be made both by professionals and patients. The prescription process for these forms of treatment often takes place in a context of the aftermath of major surgery, and patients must manage the effects of such treatment while becoming committed to new treatments and treatment calendars. Preparations must be made for dealing with daily life complicated increasingly by the physical impact of treatment and the logistics of the treatment calendar. Uncertainty about exactly what will be the impact of treatment, as well as a general context of ambiguity surrounding the issue of prognosis, complicate plan-making for the patient and family.

Once the diagnosis was made, the work of adjusting daily life to accommodate the proposed treatment calendar began in earnest. For those patients with radical courses of radiotherapy of four to six weeks, the prospect of getting to and from daily treatment was daunting. Patients with chemotherapy schedules in addition to radiotherapy, who lived in or near City B, were occasionally administered their chemotherapy at a City B hospital for their convenience. Patients who did not drive or own cars were reliant on either the ambulance or on family or friends for lifts. Reliance on the ambulance could extend the treatment day by four to seven hours for those living outside City A, and by one to three hours for local residents.

Vague boundaries exist between the work of the early illness calendar and the point at which a diagnosis is given, and between the diagnosis and the start of the treatment calendar; vague boundaries between phases typify the cancer illness calendar. Instituting the treatment calendar can be a difficult process, involving resource availability; set-up time; coordination of dates and schedules for one aspect of the calendar in one institution or department with those of another; coordination of different professionals; and the transfer of information from departments and institutions. The expenditure of resources, such as time, and those of physical energy and attention (mental and emotional energy), forms a basic condition of the treatment experience. This condition, it is argued here, touches on key issues in the quality of care (and thus, the quality of life) of cancer patients in treatment.

One of the central features of the cancer treatment calendar is the lack of choice the patient has in its detail. Short of refusing to enter a treatment calendar, or of choosing to 'drop out' of one in progress, patients are routinely presented with treatment plans as imperatives (not possibilities), or as *'faits accompli'*, over which they have no control. Going against the wishes of powerful professionals is at the very least daunting, and in doing so, the patient runs the risk of alienating those most central to treatment. Here Anita, 72, a retired mineral water company manager, describes her opposition to radiotherapy following extensive surgery for floor-of-mouth cancer:

AR: They asked me then, or rather they told me, that I would need radiotherapy. They all meet together, I think it's once a week. And I went in – poor Dr D! [radiotherapy consultant]. *He* was the one who had to tell me. You see *C* didn't and *B* didn't [hospital consultant and surgeon]. I think they *knew* I was going to be disappointed. So it was left to Dr D and he did it very well. I said, 'I'm not having *anything* done at *all*, for some little time,' I said, 'I've had quite enough' . . . He said, 'Well, how long is a little while?' I said, 'Oh, two or three weeks.' He said, 'Not two or three *months*, oh all right then.' Because *he* is the only person who's actually done what he *said* he'd do, he said he'd *write* to me doctor. Both the others, C and B, said they'd write to the GP, now Dr D *did* . . . I don't suppose anybody, had ever *dared* to uh, say, 'No I'm sorry I'm not going to have anything further done, for a little while', in a big meeting like that with all these doctors. But I've been a manager all my life, and once you've had that courage it never leaves you. Only a person with my experience could do it, an ordinary person couldn't have.

Sandelowski and Corson Jones (1996), in a paper about parents' 'choice' of prenatal diagnosis, point out that there are several different 'emplotments of choice' at work in such situations, and these can also be seen to have relevance for choice in the cancer treatment context. They describe the 'cultural story' of expanded choice arising out of the ruling interests of technological Western medicine, and the 'counter-cultural story' which shows this expanded choice to be a fiction. In the case of persons with cancer, both the 'hi-tech' nature of medical treatment, and the continuing limitations of medical knowledge about the nature of cancers and their treatment confound the issue of 'choice' of different treatments by the patient. Knowing how to assess the efficacy of different treatment approaches can be impossible for patients without specialist knowledge.

Learning about the post-surgical treatment calendar was described as a 'shock' by many patients, as in most cases little mention of adjuvant therapy had been made earlier in the illness calendar. Post-surgical patients described their disappointment over learning that they were to have lengthy schedules of radiotherapy and/or chemotherapy in addition to their surgeries. Adam, 58, a retired textile worker with lung cancer, and his wife, describe the 'shock' of hearing about his coming radiotherapy treatment:

> *Wife:* Well he [surgeon's registrar] more or less, said, he didn't know whether Dr D would even *want* to do any treatment, because, they were reasonably certain that they'd got it all away he said, and if, you know, we're not talking about the full *blast* [radiotherapy] treatment, it would just be a mild *dose* so, fair enough I mean, you go a fortnight after and they tell you you're going to have twenty days' *treat*ment well that =
>
> *AL:* = That doctor *did* say, he didn't know length of *time*, it's the amount they give you each *time*, but yeah, it were a shock and I *told* her so.
>
> *Wife:* Well *you* thought of chemotherapy.
>
> *AL:* *I* thought he said, I thought he'd said *chemo*therapy, but Joyce didn't think he *did* so, it even came *stronger* to me, you know with her saying it'd be this [radiotherapy], like against chemotherapy.

With no context in which to place such treatment, notions of 'mild' doses, long or short calendars, and the prognostic significance of the treatment calendar are hard to interpret.

The 'effects trajectory'

The 'effects trajectory' refers to the course that the side effects of each treatment will take: when they will start, intensify, and how long they will last. It is a 'trajectory' because the precise nature of the impact of a particular treatment is an unknown at the outset of the treatment calendar for each patient, even though the range of *possible* 'side' effects is known from past use of the treatment with individuals and groups. So-called 'side' effects (non-therapeutic) are often those most directly *experienced* by patients in treatment (although swift improvements may be obtained, for example, in breathing by reducing tumour size in radiotherapy).

Post-surgical patients waiting to start adjuvant radiotherapy and/or chemotherapy were often dealing with many side effects from their surgical treatment, with little or no expressed knowledge of their healing trajectory. Here May, 53, a pub caterer with floor-of-mouth cancer describes dealing with the effects of surgery at the start of her four-week radiotherapy schedule:

> MS: It's just, I don't like this *breathing* job, or me *mouth*'s always dry, in bed at night. *No* saliva at all, *none*. If I haven't got a water at side of me bed all night. Ano*ther* thing, when I want to turn over I have to actually *sit* up, and turn over, never done *that* before. I were awakened a lot last night, I've got to sit up and then lie down when I want to, you know. Also me *jaws*. I had a fish dinner, as I thought I could chew one, and *ooh* me jaw started, and it was as though it *locks*, I'm wondering if they got hold of the jaw as well you see . . . Have you seen my arm? It's lovely to what it were, it were a right, deep hole. It's built *up*, I couldn't be*lieve* it when I saw how it had built up. When I first saw it, I thought *gosh* if I bend me wrist I'll *break* it, it were that thin you could hardly *see* owt you know what I mean, it were, it's all up *here* [pointing to face, where arm section had been sewn on after tumour removal].

With the apparent lack of a formal approach in any of the three hospitals concerned to surgical aftercare, there were problems with obtaining physiotherapy, wound care and pain control following discharge (care within hospital units was described as excellent), and with information about the trajectory of these sequelae from surgery. This picture reflects that given by Williams (1993) who describes surgical patients' marked lack of knowledge of the effects of anaesthetic and the time frame for a return to normal fitness. In addition to citing the 'passive behaviour' of patients as reason for this, Williams describes the fast and chaotic management of surgical patients as contributing to these knowledge gaps. The patients whose accounts are featured in this book were often dependent on GPs and district nurses for solutions to post-surgical problems. Melissa, 49, a university housekeeper, describes getting imaginative help for her lumpectomy wound from her GP:

> MG: So I went down to me doctor and had a word with the nurse, and whilst I was *there*, me own doctor had come into the surgery and had seen us sat in the waiting room so she asked us in to have a word with her, which I thought was really nice as we didn't have an appointment. So *she* had a look at it, and got the

nurse to dress it in a gauzy kind of thing. Then when I went back again, she said, 'I've been *think*ing what we could *put* on there,' she says, 'and I've come up with this idea.' And it looked like a piece of leather, funny-looking stuff *really* and it just sort of *stuck* over the wound. I'll tell you what though, it was marvellous stuff whatever it's *been*, because it's healed it up *beau*tiful.

Alice, 50, the owner of a soft furnishings business, describes trying to manage in hospital following her lumpectomy:

AW: When you go into hospital for this sort of operation, they never tell you that you're far better getting a nightdress that you can step into. You just, haven't *any idea* what *dead*ness, you know, it sort of, the inability to move your arm you're going to have . . . nobody *men*tions that. And, to *try* and get into a nightdress with a slight sleeve is just an impossibility. The other thing, which I jotted down, was physiotherapy, which nobody's suggested.

Lymph node removal under the arm had the effect of weakening and disabling the affected arm as well as producing wounds that needed dressing and care. The effects of Tamoxifen, a drug that blocks oestrogen, were another problem for post-surgical breast cancer patients. Effects likely to be related to the Tamoxifen included nightsweats, hot flushes, body odour, period cessation, skin dryness and discoloration (and eventually, osteoporosis). Helen, 63, a housewife with breast cancer, describes her experiences of Tamoxifen's 'side' effects while in hospital:

HB: I'm having this drug this Tamoxifen, and I wake up in the middle of the night, absolutely – well, no not so much now, wearing off a bit, in the hospital I was *drenched*, I had to have the sheets changed let alone the nightie. And uh, the staff nurse didn't, quite, you know, we wondered what on earth it was. But, I've told people about it and they've said oh *yes*, I had that during the menopause. Well *I* never had anything like that, no problems at all. And, it's cropped up *three* times I've heard this, business, about you know, sweats and, perspiration. So that'll be what it is, it's the hormone pill.

None of the women taking Tamoxifen had been given any indication that it had side effects, and none had reported any to their consultants or GPs.[1] It is likely that different treatment modes will interact to produce or exacerbate 'effects', and thus there is an even greater need for an effects trajectory projection to be made.

Having some help in interpreting the effects of surgery was heard to be very important in patients' accounts of this phase of treatment. Here Adam describes having such help from a young locum, following a series of angina attacks post-discharge from hospital, after having a lung removed:

> AL: He was quite good wasn't he, speaking from the point of view that, what me body had *gone* through and uh, through the operation he was adamant that it was, delayed action from *that*, because I wasn't doing a thing, wasn't even washing *up* then was I Jan! So I mean on the second, time that he come back I'd just had another attack, I'd had two or three that morning, and uh, that made up his mind.
>
> Wife: You see, even though we as*sume* we know all this treatment is a pre*cau*tion, *basi*cally, we *don't* know, do we?
>
> AL: No, no, we don't know whether, it's still *there*.

At the root of patients' expressed post-surgical and pre-radiotherapy anxieties was the question, still unanswerable, of what exactly had happened to the cancer. Patients asked themselves, 'Is it still there? Do I still *have* cancer?' (the medical rhetoric surrounding surgery focuses on the removal of the cancer, and casts further treatment as 'precautionary'); and, 'Which of my "effects" is related to the treatment? Which to the cancer?' (the ever-present threat of spread); 'How long will it take for me to recover from treatment?' and so forth.

Instances where the effects trajectory *had* been made explicit by a senior or 'key' professional (not a 'helper') were few. Larry, 70, a retired factory foreman with terminal lung cancer, describes a consultant's frank description of his palliative radiotherapy:

> LH: He said how it won't affect me just now, but when I go home and in a few weeks it *will*. I'll take pain in me chest, I won't be able to swallow, I'll feel like death, and then, when I get over that, it *may* make me breathe a bit easier. No guarantee.

Here a description is relayed of the effects and limitations of a treatment that is not going to be curative but which may alleviate breathing difficulty. The consultant had given Larry the idea of a trajectory – when to expect certain effects, and the *possible* benefits and drawbacks of treatment. Understanding the limits of possible side effects from treatment was also described as reassuring – learning what treatment would *not* do was also important.

Patients described the importance of knowing something in advance of how treatment modes might affect them, so that they could plan their management of these effects and any necessary alterations to the personal calendar, such as getting time off work, renewing sick notes, getting help with household tasks or child care, and finding out about support services. Betty, 44, a retired WREN with breast cancer, describes concerns about the effects trajectories of both her radiotherapy and chemotherapy treatments:

> *BG:* I won't say it's weighing heavily on my mind but once again, you're into the realms of the slightly unknown. I know the procedure, I know it's not going to hurt because I hate pain, I'm a complete coward. I know it's not going to take very long, I think the one thing is I suppose more than anything else is the chemotherapy. When he [consultant] actually said, radiation plus a course of chemotherapy, 'cause once again you've heard so many stories about the effects of chemotherapy, but reading that booklet, it doesn't affect everybody the same. You know, I think that is it at the moment, what effect is that going to have on me? . . . I'm not quite sure what the period of time for the chemotherapy, whether it's, once a week, once a, month, or whatever, but over a three-month period, that's what he said, initially. So I think that really is, the effect that's going to have on me, *how* ill am I going to be, am I still going to, you know run my home, you know, how much is it going to knock me out, so to speak.

A key issue highlighted by many patients' effects trajectory concerns is that it is not cure alone, but also the *price* (in terms of both physical impact and impact on the personal calendar) of a possible cure or disease reduction, an original goal of quality of life measurement. Dan, 76, a retired quantities surveyor with urinary tract cancer, and his wife wondered in interview if his radiotherapy treatment was 'worth it', given the strain of travel to and from the centre from City B daily and the effects of the radiotherapy. Their concern hinged upon their not having a clear prognostic picture from discussions with professionals:

> *DG:* We don't know, *what* my position is, all we know is, I've got two separate cancers, and that I'm going to be treated for them, *and* under these conditions nowadays, if it works *won*ders or what, but as to whether I'm *per*manently, or, three months, six months or a *year* to live I haven't a clue. And what I mean is, I'm one of these, whatever's going to be will *be*, and I'd rather they'd come out and just tell me, what the exact position *is* . . . Well, this is my first week, but *I* should be inclined after the *sec*ond week I'll be saying then well *look* doctor, *what* is the exact position?
>
> *Wife:* He's been really down and in bed most of the time. He's sick and really an invalid, and now I've wondered is it, *worth* him going through all that treatment if it was just for, a few more months.

Wanting to know 'what the position' was regarding prognosis was a much-cited concern, despite the fear many patients expressed about having to hear 'bad news'.

Useful effects trajectory work in the radiotherapy setting (carried out by radiographers) focused on helping patients to understand radiotherapy as distinct from chemotherapy. For surgical patients, knowing what the recovery trajectory was likely to be and how to interpret pain were key issues. Patients for whom surgery had meant permanent losses of function needed help in managing these and advice on how future treatment would affect them. Others with existing chronic conditions needed to know how treatment for cancer would affect them, and how it might interact with medications they were already taking. These concerns were largely neglected in the treatment context.

In making frequent references to the 'individualism' of the *patient's* reaction to treatment, calendar professionals were already setting the stage for treatment as a mysterious and unaccountable process beyond querying by the patient. Much that was to have a direct bearing on patients' functioning in the future was discounted. The issue of the limitations of treatment and medical knowledge, as well as that of choice in treatment are excluded from discussions of treatment with patients within an individualistic, biomedical perspective. Lack of detailed attention to effects trajectory issues is a part of this obscuring of awareness (whether intentional or not) of the deeper issues of treatment and medicalized illness.

Location in the treatment calendar: vague boundaries

It is a simple but frequently overlooked point in the literature on chronic illness that treatment calendars are *not* always neatly laid out, linear, or 'fixed' in shape. The treatment calendar can be a very 'fuzzy' entity, subject to all sorts of difficulties with set-up, stalls, gaps during, and sudden alteration along its course. Even when on course, treatment proper may take time to get under way. Here Ellie, 64, a retired catering assistant, discusses this situation:

> ER: I'm going on Friday for my first treatment . . . you see this is another thing. You see, well, you don't know, you just think, three weeks' treatment starts on Monday but you see *Mon*day I went to have all the marks and everything done, and I thought right, *Tues*day I start the treatment, but you see, it doesn't work like that 'cause they have it all to work out filling the position in of the x-rays or something, so I don't start while Friday!

Abby, 46, an ex-nurse and NHS manager, and a gestalt therapist at the time of her diagnosis of recurrent multi-focal breast cancer, remarks on the same 'information gap' regarding the treatment calendar:

AW: That was a distinct gap in information which actually threw me because I had to ring round all my clients and re-organize them, because, being given my *first* appointment for November 12, and being told yeah, you go then, November 12, and you then have 20 days' treatment so I sort of worked out, excluding Saturdays and Sundays, and, I wished I'd been told, well you *go* on that day, *but* it will be several days before you start treatment and we won't know how many days. So I'm at *least* given an idea of well, it could be, or it could be longer. And I thought yeah, this has set me *back* a week . . . They really need to *say* to patients, yeah you will come to prescription clinic and you will not start treatment until all the, making of the shields and what have you is ready, and that will not happen until a week later.

Respect for the demands of patients' personal calendars seemed lacking in the lack of information they were given about the centre's own implicit schedules. For patients with two treatment calendars in addition to surgical follow-up, management of the personal calendar was especially complex. Betty, 44, a retired WREN working part-time as a cleaner at a local hotel, describes orienting herself to both her radiotherapy and chemotherapy calendars:

BG: I mean, at the moment I'm thinking I'm in the five weeks at [City A], that's how far I've got up to at the moment. I know I've got to go every day nine o'clock in the morning for five days a week, and then when I know the chemotherapy I'll be that further on and then it will be, you know I'll be looking a*head* then working out right *that* will be the last time, and then we take it from there. But obviously I'm thinking long-term I mean, March, April next year? Easter-time? Hopefully by then, finished you know, clear, obviously reviews then at such and such a time, you know once a month once every six months, a year, or whatever.

Betty describes the start of the chemotherapy schedule as a marker in the treatment calendar, its uncertain finish pointing to the future of reviews which will comprise the post-treatment illness calendar (always containing the possibility of recurrence or spread, and more treatment). As yet, Betty does not know the detail of the chemotherapy schedule (or indeed, what effect the two treatment modes will have on her ability to function in the personal calendar), or the pattern of review after treatment, so much of the treatment calendar remains nebulous, unfixable to points in the calendar year ahead. The importance of daily orientation within the treatment calendar was a regular theme in respondents' accounts of treatment at this preparation stage. Betty continues:

BG: I . . . I've lived on my own, the problems of owning a home and
problems of, driving from A to B or, the problems of overseas
living, serving overseas, just, doing things quietly and method-
ically thinking things *out*, knowing where, right, I've got an
appointment at [City A] for nine o'clock on Friday morning,
what time do I leave, what time do I get up? I mean, these are
the things that are important to me, because I know *who* I am
exactly with, you know you coming this morning or, I'll do that
and that, and at such-and-such a time.

What might be called the 'cracked idiom', 'knowing *who* I am exactly',
underscores the primacy of the calendar in Western culture. Suggested here
is that location in the calendar is a matter of identity; Betty is in some
ways a different person when she is interviewed in her home than when
she is a patient keeping an appointment at the centre, or when she is doing
errands in the village. Ezzy (1993) describes the centrality of 'life-plans'
or 'strategies for interaction' in identity theory. Such plans are necessary
to provide a 'stable, dependable source of identity legitimation – typically
through the establishment of routines and patterned interaction with significant others' (1993: 49–50). The treatment calendar necessitates the forming
of new life-plans because of its impact on the personal calendars of patients.
Continuity within the treatment calendar is contingent on regular contact
with the same people within established routines. Locating oneself within
the treatment calendar is a first step to taking up the threads of one's personal
calendar again, following a diagnosis of cancer.

Treatment calendars can be subject to change, particularly when there
are multiple treatment options available. Here Rachael, 41, a supply teacher
with breast cancer, describes preparations for her post-lumpectomy radiotherapy treatment calendar:

RS: I did get a shock *there*, because I've now been informed that
because the, *cut* is close to the cancerous *cells* that I'm going to
have to go into [the centre] for, well four days *after* my radiotherapy as an in-patient, to have some, rods inserted, which is
just an added precaution. So I'm just getting over the shock of
having to go back in really. Although, you know it's *no* problem
it's just a, an extension of, because I don't *feel* ill it just seems a,
pro*long*ing, me getting back to, normal, life and you know, as a
sup*ply* teacher I enjoyed it and, we were going on a holiday, we
had to cancel our holiday, which was a bit disappointing. We
were going to America . . . So it's a good job that I'd, we *did*
cancel because what with having to go into [the centre] again as
an in-patient, we won't, know where *would* I have been really.
I doubt I'd be ready to go, it would *clash* anyway.

Despite the minimization of treatment as 'precautionary', Rachael describes the news as a 'shock', perhaps because it could indicate a more serious disease situation (treatment calendars are, in their detail, the main and often sole source of information for patients about prognosis). The news is described as a shock because of the prolongation of the treatment and illness calendars (despite Rachael not feeling 'ill') and subsequent delay and cancellation of events in the personal calendar.

The ability to locate oneself within the treatment calendar has practical implications for the personal calendar, as described by Betty below:

> BG: You see my sick note expires on the 3rd of December, so by the time . . . I will go and see my GP a couple of days before that, that will be after I've finished at [City A] then I will know then I should see, *how* often I'm *hav*ing the chemotherapy, what effect at the time it's having on *me*, physically and, you know, assessing then whether . . .
>
> KCS: You're going back to work?
>
> BG: Oh yeah I would pre*fer* to go back to work because it . . . I . . . I'm *do*ing something, I'm one of these persons that likes to *do* . . . be on the go all the time I get, you get *bored* . . . and the hotel I work at are very good, they're absolutely smashing you know, and I only work three hours a day. I work six days, and have one day off. Well I could start just going in for three or four days three or four mornings, well, you know.

Here Betty describes the interdependence of the two calendars. The expiry of the sick note follows close on the heels of the end of radiotherapy, necessitating a trip to the GP and a decision: whether or not to renew the note or return to work. Renewing the note would prolong 'patienthood' and returning to work is both a matter of identity *and* economy. This decision depends on her (as yet unknown) response to the chemotherapy, and to the interaction of the radiotherapy and the chemotherapy effects. The sick note covers the radiotherapy period but not the (as yet undecided) chemotherapy schedule. The vagueness of *when* the missing information will be known, combined with the other details discussed, evokes the 'limbo' of treatment calendar preparation, a nebulousness and uncertainty that will hang over the eventual calendar throughout its course, and beyond it to review. The latter unknown future illness calendar is discussed by Helen, 63, a housewife with breast cancer:

> HB: I haven't been told, officially, how often I'll go, I'll be called back, or if I will in*deed* be called back. Whether you have a, pattern after you finish maybe you talk to, I've to see Mr Y [the surgeon] again, and, when the uh, treatment's over I haven't got a date for that yet but in the middle of the treatment and I asked

them on Monday what I should *do* about this appointment, so I won't lose any treatment time.

The first *surgical* review will occur in the midst of the radiotherapy schedule, and the second after it has finished. Managing surgical review appointments in such a way as not to 'lose treatment time' was an expressed concern for many patients. There was a great deal of acknowledged uncertainty over the 'pattern' of the future illness calendar, and who would preside over it.

The logistics of the treatment calendar: the impact on the personal calendar

Relatives were described as an invaluable resource in the running of the treatment calendar; getting information; confirming what was remembered of interactions with professionals; liaising on the telephone with staff; following up arrangements to ensure they were carried out; making appointments; and resolving calendar conflicts. They also provided transportation, companionship and nursing care. Their 'spokesperson' role extended to the community, friends and neighbours. Here Adam's wife describes her experience as contact person:

> *Wife:* I . . . it's *tell*ing people as *well*, and, and you see if you've *got* lots of friends re*peat*ing it over and over again to people you know that they will ask and that, *that* was uh, got me upset. And you know if we were to, it would have been easier to put a thing through the newspaper and, heh heh, let people know without asking!

Travelling to and from treatment was no small part of the daily calendar, as Nina, 61, a housewife with breast cancer describes:

> *NS:* Well yes that's going to be, with it, like a job really. But fortunately my husband's re*tir*ed so he can take me. Of course it's the, what three-quarters of an hour *jour*ney each way! Huh for what uh, about *ten* minutes of treatment or something like that! It's a great pity they haven't got any equipment in [City B], but uh, of course it's a specialist *treat*ment and they have all their everything at [City A], so that's it.

Francesca, 67, a widowed housewife with thigh sarcoma describes arranging with family for a ride to the centre for daily treatment:

> *FA:* Me granddaughter's taking me up today again. I've had family take me, up to *now* and, and then me youngest granddaughter she goes to [a college in a town some distance from City A], but

Monday Tuesday and Wednesday she finishes by lunchtime so she's going to take me up those three days. And then I have some friends that are going to fit other days in, to take me up. But eventually afterwards, I'm hoping I can just go up on bus meself because it's only about three stops up the *road*, you know. It's better than waiting for ambulances! You never know when they're coming! ... Last time I went down to the [diagnosing hospital in City A] in ambulance, when I had to see Dr X [consultant at centre], took us three-quarters of an hour to go there heh! We went to collect five people and we only picked up two, three weren't coming!

Even with local residence, keeping to the treatment calendar was described as hard work for patients and a network of relatives and friends. Patients required their own means of transport, or that provided by close others, in order to maintain any control over their own time each weekday. The freedom to control one's own time might be considered a central aspect of 'quality of life' in the treatment calendar.

The treatment calendar is dependent on the absence of small disasters, like machine breakdown (radiotherapy), and on the availability of professionals (in cases where treatment is given outside the centre, in special clinics run by centre staff), and of information (such as blood counts, x-rays, histology reports). There are threats to the personal calendar (both the daily calendar and the 'life calendar') implicit in treatment, in the treatment calendar and its organization, and in the treatment context, with its organizational difficulties. For the cancer patient beginning treatment, these threats perhaps comprise the central threat to 'quality of life' posed by the illness.

The cancellation or suspension of plans is not only an initial condition of the treatment calendar, but becomes a steady feature of the personal calendar. Here Ellie describes not being able to commit herself to activities outside the treatment calendar with certainty:

ER: I don't want to talk about it really I don't, because it, I mean it's *there* all the time anyway I'd love to get it, finished with and get *on* with me, with me *life* you know and get on with other things, but at the moment it's all *this*, 'cause it's there all the time ... although as I say I haven't been *ill* or anything. But if you're playing in a team and you feel oh I might, if I don't feel like playing on Wednesday I might let them down, you see I won't bother.

The pervasiveness of the treatment calendar and the sense of living in suspended animation is evoked by Ellie in this excerpt. Often, the newly-diagnosed person in treatment does not feel 'ill' but cannot live like a well person because they cannot be fully dependable in the personal calendar. Plan-making must be suspended, and the loss of 'dependability' means temporary losses in the personal calendar for many patients. This lack of dependability had serious consequences for those whose livelihood rested on plan-making and honouring. Here Jim, 63, a saw operator with cancer of the bladder, talks about the difficulty of managing work during diagnosis and treatment schedule set-up:

> JW: . . . I missed *this* week though. I'm going to try and get a sick note to cover me for the *week*.
> KCS: Is that proving difficult for you?
> JW: I don't *know* whether that's all, *well* I'll go to me own GP if they won't give me one any other way. But they should give me one they're *talk*ing in the region of two *months*, so a month's treatment and another month before I'm fit to go back to *work*.

Jim's work is paid by the hour, and he receives no pay for time off. Lack of a bus route to his remote village meant he drove himself to and from the treatment centre – a total of 1600 miles during a single month of treatment. The uncertainty of his position is underscored in this excerpt:

> JW: Well *that's* the hardest thing it's uh, it's trying to get enough work to make a living. I mean I could have done with another two or three weeks at work and I'd have been *home* free.
> KCS: Are you thinking of coming in [as an in-patient] eventually before the =
> JW: = *No* I won't come in. I was just talking to a chap in there he says he's had, 16 visits now and *he's* driving himself. But he says he's, he lives at [a village near City A] and he's having no problems, so if *he* can I can.

Personal calendar losses consitute losses, temporary or permanent, or repeated, of identity-in-the-social-world for the person. Even (perhaps especially) in the case of dying patients whose personal calendars are ultimately threatened in the face of death the personal calendar continues to be important, though it may have a very limited space within a context increasingly dominated by illness and treatment. Here Gary, 60, a plumber with mesothelioma (asbestos cancer), discusses a moment during an at-home examination:

> GL: There was a *hawk* landing in them evergreen shrubs and that was when the doctor from the health service *came* here to examine me. Well he was stood there and I was laid here, and I just glanced round while he was talking to me, I couldn't be*lieve* it, I said, 'Look at that doctor!'

KCS: Would it ever try to get at your birds?

GL: Well I haven't seen any doing it. I think they're starting to nest now so I'm hoping, I've got me fingers crossed. I'm hoping to breed off 'em.

There is a kind of parallel discourse here: the hopelessness of a certain and very difficult death from an especially intractable form of cancer, and the continued interest in living, expressed in the making of plans. Both are equally present in this excerpt, not contradictory. The personal calendar, no matter how constrained, encompasses much that is central to personal and social identity. The illness calendar/treatment calendar displaces the personal calendar to an extent (frequently to a large extent), and this constitutes a form of suffering for the ill person.

For several patients, treatment meant incurring losses in addition to the loss of time that had serious repercussions for the personal and life calendars. Here Alice, 50, describes being unable to work actively in her soft furnishings business on account of her loss of arm strength and mobility from a lumpectomy and removal of lymph nodes:

AW: There is *no way* that I can do the job that is *mine*, in the business, because of me arm, there's just no way that I can do it, 'cause it's extremely *heavy*, you know I can be throwing a velvet curtain about that's got five widths in them, they're extremely *heavy*, there's no way I can do it. And I *need* to be able to stretch. Until I . . . there's no way the, arm is too painful, to even do it *once*, you know. And really, that's all that, *both*ers me is that, I will no longer be able to do the job that I would be doing. But I'm not *e*motional about it 'cause I've done it for so long. We'll *find* somebody else that's *a*ble to do it and we'll just have to chuck off and get *on* with it.

The loss of mobility (and the lengthy radiation and chemotherapy schedules facing her) entail the loss, at least temporarily, of Alice's *role* in her business, and pose a potential threat to her livelihood (if the loss proves not to be temporary). The importance of additional therapies (like physiotherapy) in the managing of treatment's 'side' effects must be emphasized here, as the true cost of treatment will be experienced in these 'side' effects. Not being able any longer to 'do the job that I would be doing . . . for so long' is a real threat posed by treatment:

KCS: Will you be involved in running the business still, or . . .

AW: But I've lost my *role*, I would have to *find* another *role* that I was *happy* with, the role that I *had* you know what I mean 'cause i— it was my *baby*. I was the only one that knew anything about the business although I had a partner, she's sort of just drifted along with the *tide*, and the business has grown *with* us, so she can cope with the selling part in the shop. But I for the *minu*te I've just lost my *role*, my *cen*tre, and th— the certainness of [things] because, if they don't do as *I* say, without me there isn't a *busi*ness.

These losses, potential or already fact, entail among other things the loss of 'certainness' (or what might be termed a calendar loss), and there is tension in this excerpt between this loss as being 'for the minute' only, and its possible permanence, with major implications for Alice's personal and life calendars.

Alice goes on to contrast the loss of her role with the loss of breast tissue through lumpectomy:

AW: I don't feel emotional about having lost off a *boob* because, there was never a great deal there in the *first* place! [laughs] so, uhm, I . . . I *feel* that me boobs weren't an asset so I've . . . I've lived with*out* them all this time! It didn't . . . it didn't matter, but uhm, I like to keep something happening, such as sort of going out *some*where. I *can't* just sit here, I've *got* to get inv*olv*ed with things. Sort of keep an eye on the business and try to think of another *angle* for bringing money in. I've got to keep me mind on it to keep *from* sinking into, you know the *slight*est depression I don't want that to happen. Uh, although I've been *war*ned that with, radium, that *does* happen.

The loss of breast tissue is described as not a real loss because 'I've lived with*out* them all this time!' The loss of her work, however, means a loss of 'somewhere' to go each day, 'something happening', and being 'involved with things' that must be replaced by a new personal and daily calendar, 'another angle for bringing money in' being a part of this new calendar. The implementation of a new calendar (dealing with the losses incurred through treatment and the treatment calendar) is thus identified as a practical matter for Alice, as well as a matter of identity, and finally, as a matter of dealing with the effects of treatment – the need to keep from 'sinking into . . . depression', a possible consequence of radiotherapy.

The treatment calendar (including potential effects of treatment and their trajectories) effectively blocks access to the personal calendar, a process begun at the start of the illness calendar. The reduction in 'lifespace' is dimensional – different people are socially involved to different extents. The uncertainty attending this threat to the personal calendar by the illness and treatment calendars – 'How much will I have to give up? For how long?' – is a way of conceptualizing the much-cited uncertainty attending the experience of cancer and its treatment.

Box 4.1: *Summary of treatment calendar problems*

There were many problems with treatment calendar management described by patients. Treatment calendars were often dogged by interaction problems, schedule hold-ups, misinformation and lack of liaison. Below is a summary of general types of problems experienced by some of the patients whose stories are featured elsewhere in this book.

1 Ellie, 64, a retired catering assistant with breast cancer, was mistaken for another patient (who had had a radical mastectomy) by her surgeon during recovery from lumpectomy, and was told she was not to have any further treatment; when the mistake was rectified, she was told instead that she would have three weeks' outpatient radiotherapy and four days' radioactive wire implant treatment, and decided that this meant her prognosis was much worse than the other woman's.

2 Phil, 58, a retired bait farm worker and angler with lung cancer, experienced diagnostic confusion over the nature of the diagnosis and treatment options (given several conflicting assessments of operability). Diagnosis and prognostic information was delivered by junior doctors, with the consultant failing to appear at pre-arranged times to discuss these with Phil. He was referred for palliative radiotherapy without first receiving a definitive statement about diagnosis or prognosis until he 'pulled up' the two juniors and insisted they tell him.

3 Bronwyn, 58, a housewife with cancer of the chortoid (part of the eye), was under care privately for cataracts in her eye (she had hoped to avoid the two-year waiting list for cataract removal). She had planned a three-month visit to Australia prior to seeing the consultant. He then refused to operate until she had returned from abroad. The day before she was to leave, she was rushed to hospital and a large chortoid tumour was detected attached to the eye. Bronwyn and her husband said that no diagnosis of cancer was communicated to either of them, and her husband was unable to locate any of the professionals involved to question them as to the precise nature of the diagnosis after Bronwyn had been admitted to hospital. Once in radiotherapy, the original private consultant sent her an appointment card to have the cataracts in her now-missing eye removed. Her regular GP on a home visit asked her if she had any sight left in it (she changed to another practice after this).

4 May, 53, a pub caterer with floor-of-mouth cancer, had been fitted by her dentist with dentures, which began to be uncomfortable two months afterwards. The dentist filed down the dentures after a second consultation, but did not look in May's mouth at the time. After four more months, she consulted him again with extreme pain and inability to wear the dentures, during which he again suggested filing. She asked for an examination and he then noticed the tumour. May reported that no clear diagnosis (of *cancer*) was given to her or her husband. Later her radiotherapy consultant explained to students in her presence that the cancer had gone 'very

deep' and was more extensive than previously thought, details she had not been told before.

5 Kevin, 60, a former security officer, actually had leukaemia at the time of his diagnosis with floor-of-mouth cancer, though he was unaware of this. He was 'diagnosed' when his GP read a letter sent by the consultant who had diagnosed him with floor-of-mouth cancer, in which mention was made of his leukaemia (an earlier letter from the leukaemia consultant – whom Kevin had seen for what he thought was a 'blood imbalance' – had been sent to another GP in the practice by mistake, so neither Kevin nor his GP knew about the leukaemia until the second letter was read).

Kevin had agreed to be entered into a clinical trial of a new radiotherapy regimen at the centre, but the professionals in charge of it had not been made aware of Kevin's leukaemia diagnosis, which disqualified him from entry. The resulting change in Kevin's treatment calendar when the mistake was found out meant that his treatment start was delayed by ten days, during which no communication was made by the centre to Kevin as to when treatment would start.

6 Adam, 58, a retired textiles worker with lung cancer, was referred by the first consultant he saw to another consultant after 'spots on the lung' had been discovered in x-rays. This consultant presumed the first had diagnosed these as malignant, so Adam was 'diagnosed' only when the second consultant referred to his having extensive malignancies requiring removal of the lung (Adam did not recall the word 'cancer' as mentioned by either consultant). Adam described persistent problems with information from the two key professionals involved at this stage, including two conflicting assessments of operability. He was not told about his extensive radiotherapy calendar until after the operation for removal of his affected lung. Adam was discharged from hospital following his operation without pain medication. He was readmitted by a locum following an attack of his long-standing angina.

7 Alice, 50, a soft furnishings business owner with breast cancer, consulted her GP with a breast lump in January, which her GP insisted was benign and needed no follow-up. She was finally referred in October for a D and C. At this time, she was sent to a surgeon for a breast biopsy, the results of which were negative. The operation for removal of the lump was booked but postponed for three and a half months because of changes in hospital organization, and took place in January of the following year. Four weeks later, Alice was recalled for a diagnosis of cancer and further biopsies, but no account for the delay was communicated to her. Two weeks later she had a second operation to remove lymph glands in her arm. She required physiotherapy for her arm, but was only referred when she 'pressed' the radiotherapy consultant for a referral, three months after the second operation.

8 Rachael, 41, a supply teacher with breast cancer, had negative biopsy results which conflicted with the histological report post-lumpectomy, and this contradiction was never addressed directly by the consultant. Neither

Rachael nor her husband could recall the word 'cancer' being used by any professional involved. There was no liaison between the hospital and Rachael's husband, such that he 'lost track' of her temporarily following a second operation to remove lymph glands. Rachael was given conflicting information about further treatment by the surgeon and his senior registrar, and the confusion was not resolved until she arrived at the centre for radiotherapy and was informed of her prescribed treatment.

Rachael had had chemotherapy administered to her at City B hospital by an unsupervised houseman resulting in a large wound in her hand that was thought by the radiotherapy consultant to warrant plastic surgery afterwards. No follow-up care was provided for the wound. (Problems with chemotherapy at this hospital were experienced by all three women interviewed who had post-surgical chemotherapy, because of a lack of regular set-up for its administration, and administration by junior, unsupervised staff. This was later rectified by the appointment of a chemotherapy nurse at the hospital.)

9 Terry, 64, a retired electronics technician with larynx cancer, was not referred to a consultant even after his GP had given him three courses of antibiotics over a four-week period, forcing Terry to 'go private' for a diagnosis of the lump in his throat. Terry said that there had been no mention of the word 'cancer' by the diagnosing consultant at diagnosis (he was told he had a 'malignant growth' instead). Terry was inappropriately entered onto a clinical trial at the treatment centre (he had a heart condition that should have disqualified him). He requested release from the trial after he was told he would not start treatment for five weeks, owing to his having 'missed' the current round of randomization. He was having trouble breathing and speaking caused by a tumour on his larynx (surgery was not possible because of his heart condition) and he felt he could not wait for treatment. Being dropped from the trial delayed the start of radiotherapy for two weeks.

Treatment calendar professionals

The major investment of senior treatment professionals (surgeons, consultants and their registrars) in terms of time and expertise is made before the start of the post-surgical treatment calendar, in the work of diagnosis, surgery if possible, the provision of a treatment trajectory and the prescription of radiotherapy and/or chemotherapy courses. Once the treatment calendar is embarked upon, most of the work of *treating* is done by lower status professionals (such as radiographers and nurses) who administer treatment and provide care for side effects. However, overall responsibility for the treatment *calendar* (the shape of the treatment plan) remains the province of higher status professionals.

The post-operative treatment calendar was managed by senior professionals (consultants and senior registrars) at the treatment centre, although there were also important follow-up appointments with surgeons (most usually taken by their registrars) at the two referring hospitals. Patients saw many of the same professionals as they went through the surgical and radiotherapy treatment calendars: each patient was 'under' a senior treatment professional and senior registrar in each of these treatment calendars (though many patients saw only the senior registrars or others). Senior professionals' management of the treatment calendar consisted of weekly reviews during radiotherapy, followed by a succession of reviews held at longer intervals. There was a review at one month following completion of the radiotherapy calendar, then another one to two months after this. Surgical reviews were at two to three months post-operatively. In addition, some patients had scans, biopsies and x-rays alongside treatment. All of these professionals and schedules (treatment, surveillance and follow-up) are part of the cancer illness calendar, although the dominant calendar was the radiotherapy calendar at the centre.

A main theme of this book is the 'quality of care' dimension in patients' experience of diagnosis and treatment, conceptualized in terms of professionals' treatment calendar management. Both 'key' professionals (those with the greatest status hierarchically, but also those with the greatest influence over each individual's treatment calendar), and 'helpers in the trajectory' (lower status professionals carrying out the directives of senior treatment managers) are engaged in treatment calendar management. Management of the treatment calendar involves the administering of treatment, the managing of daily treatment and 'surveillance' schedules, and the overseeing of the whole treatment calendar, as it manifests the treatment trajectories of senior treatment managers.

Locating professionals in the treatment calendar

Locating professionals in the context of the developing treatment calendar was heard to be an important task for patients. Many patients had reviews in both the post-surgical and radiotherapy/chemotherapy calendars with both consultants and their senior registrars, sometimes separately, sometimes together. Those who routinely saw the senior registrar expressed confusion over why they were 'under' a consultant they never or rarely saw, what the reasons for this were, and who the treatment *manager* was supposed to be (they described *experiencing* management from the registrar, but 'on the card' they were under the care of the consultant). Here Nina, 61, a housewife with breast cancer, voices some of this confusion:

> NS: Well that's a point – I've never *seen* Dr D [consultant at centre]
> yet! Dr L [senior registrar] the lady doctor, yes that was who I
> saw. Heh heh! I've never seen Dr D at *all*. He did come into the
> room once when I was laid out on that simulator, just to check
> something but I . . . I couldn't move and I couldn't see him, he
> was around the corner . . . I've never met him, no, which seems
> peculiar. I don't know whether I shall see him at [the referring]
> hospital, I don't know. I'm *un*der him it's on the *card*, yes. Prob-
> ably shall or not, remains to be seen I s'pose.

Not knowing 'who is in charge' can and indeed had seemed to affect
how and whether patients revealed information about their conditions, or
problems with treatment. Kevin, 60, an unemployed security guard with
floor-of-mouth cancer and leukaemia describes tearfully how an initial consultation went with the centre's dietitian at the start of his radiotherapy
course:

> KC: I had words with the dietitian when I first went to [the centre] as
> an outpatient, and I'm afraid I was a bit, not, *an*gry but, a bit
> rude I think. It sounded worse than what I intended it to do, but
> when you're losing your voice as I was at the time, it sounded
> worse than what I intended it, and I was going to ask *him* [the
> consultant] stuff. I think she took it, I've always had to be in a
> position that I had to be in con*trol*, and I thought I was in
> control. She knew I damn well *was*n't and I wasn't *going* to be,
> and she had tried to advise me and I wanted none of it. I don't
> never dare speak to her now.

In this excerpt, Kevin describes trying to take control of the situation (one
which was beginning to be 'out of control' as suggested by the loss of his
voice) which for him at this stage meant speaking to 'the one in charge'.
Knowledge of who is the central treatment calendar manager, and the role
of lower status staff in the running of the work of the treatment calendar,
was heard to be a main feature in the construction of security and continuity in the treatment calendar.

There was much discussion in interviews about 'who was who', and
who was in charge of what information. Unsurprisingly, people with previous illness histories or professional connections with hospitals (several
patients were or had been health professionals themselves) were more
accurate at locating professionals according to rank and function within
the treatment calendar. These people also described excellent management
from key professionals and 'helpers' alike, an apparent consequence of
their 'insider' status. Liam, 73, a retired dental technician and 15-year
cancer survivor with a recurrence of larynx cancer, recalls his aftercare

from an initial surgery for his first diagnosis, while still on the staff of a dental hospital in City A:

> LC: Dr F, he's retired now, he said, 'Look, you *work* at the dental hospital, it's half an hour off for you, put on your white coat', I had a white coat, and . . . it was so *han*dy you see. I think a *nor*mal person would have had an appointment say, every month, but he just wanted to make absolutely *sure*. And they did such a good job that I was on view to the students . . . and with being on the job as it were, I wouldn't say I was a guinea pig for them all, but, if they wanted to explain anything, I was the chap they could get in a minute's notice.

Betty, 44, a retired WREN with breast cancer, describes her care as a continuation of her experience with a benign breast lump the year preceding her diagnosis with cancer:

> BG: There's Mr H who is the consultant who actually, I'd seen last year and I'd also been referred to this year, uh, and he's the surgeon. Plus his resident who saw me initially and then called Mr H in to say, you know, which he confirmed and then I had dealings with a *jun*ior doctor who was doing all the questions, similar to that I had blood tests and things like that. It was just really the main two, Mr H and his resident.

Some patients found the range of players harder to locate, particularly where there was no prior illness experience from which to draw. Todd, a scaffolder with floor-of-mouth cancer, lists the professionals involved in his diagnosis:

> TA: Well I saw the specialist at the *den*tist she was the first one I saw. And I had to go to, the dental school. I saw that gentleman again, and he fetched another chap in. There was Dr C [surgeon] and the other and whether he was a registrar there or . . . he had inspected me mouth and said something to this, other gentleman so, and then he told me it was really bad, and that was when I saw Dr C and he told me what I'd got.

The names and specific positions of lower status professionals were described as rarely expressly conveyed (quoted introductions were 'I am Mr X's associate/assistant/working with Mr X' etc. to signify lower status), further complicating the task of location. Rachael, 41, a supply teacher with breast cancer, saw many professionals during her hospital stay:

> RS: Yes I'm not quite sure about, who was who. He's Doc— the one that seemed to be in charge, is it Dr C? Something like that he was, *he* seemed to be in charge and then, the *lady* doctor came

round to see me before my operation to mark me up. Right, so she marked me up, that's the same one that did my injections. But Mr H [the surgeon] came round the following morning and *did* actually say well she hadn't, marked me up properly, she should have, done *two* arrows, instead of just one pointing down, so he re-marked me.

Patients in hospital are routinely 'seen' and 'handled' by staff (often junior) of whose status they are often unaware. Meredith (1993) reports in a study of consent on a general surgery ward that over two-thirds of patients had not had the consent form explained to them, and over half did not know the status of the doctor requesting the signature. It emerged that house officers were those obtaining consent as part of their routine work, but that they were not familiar with the details of the 'treatment plans' of patients.

Problems did arise for some patients who were passed back and forth between the consultant and registrar, in terms of conflicting information about treatment, disease status and treatment trajectory, and because the capacity to form a relationship with a central treatment professional was undermined. Samantha, 36, a housewife with breast cancer, relates an incident in which her 'case' had 'suddenly' appeared to have been taken over by a registrar she had never seen before at the centre, who had related information that conflicted with the treatment plan as described by the radiotherapy consultant:

SV: He [senior registrar] never seen my report or anything I mean he's mentioning chemo*ther*apy. You know, and he never even, you know sees me report, but yet he's telling me about you know, chemotherapy on top of me radiotherapy. So then I got all upset again didn't I, you know telling you one thing and then another doctor's telling me another so I'm getting, confused. But Dr D [consultant] says I didn't have to have it, so I'm going by him, you know 'cause he's *un*der Dr D, you know. As far as I know he is.

Van der Waal *et al.* (1996), in their comparison of preference between medical specialists and patients with chronic illness, found 'continuity of care (always seeing the same doctor)' to be 'one of the most important aspects of the quality of care' for those with a chronic illness, while it remained a matter of lower priority for health care providers. Many patients expressed surprise over discovering that the treatment calendar could suddenly be seen to be in 'someone else's' hands, and that it could be changed without notice, new modes added, schedules lengthened or shortened. When the task of relaying this (often threatening and difficult to hear) information was given over to professionals the patient had never seen before, and/or there was confusion about what the 'real story' was, treatment could suddenly appear chaotic. Patients wondered aloud about what such changes could mean in terms of 'seriousness' (the question of 'how ill am I really?'). Here Bertha, 62, a retired clerk with a recurrent breast cancer, voices concerns about the meaning of subtle changes in her post-radiation treatment calendar as she is passed from person to person, that seem to suggest her cancer may have metastasized:

> BB: If you go [to the referring hospital] on a Thursday you don't see Mr H [surgeon], if you go on a Tuesday, you *do*. Well I went last time it was a young lady. Now, she's very *nice*, but I don't think she was as experienced as she might have been shall we say. 'Cause she . . . all she did was she bent me leg up and felt all round and she said she didn't think it [pain in leg] was anything to *do* with this [the cancer]. I was on six-monthly appointments then. She says 'I'll put you on three monthly then and we'll see how it's going.' Well when I went back, it was the same young man as I saw *yesterday*, he's quite nice and seems quite thorough. Well, he sent me for a bone scan. And, as I said to Dr *P* [GP] once, I said, 'You know, I'm getting a bit worried,' I said, 'because, I know that uh, cancer of the spine is a common secondary one to this', he said, 'That's what you're on Tamoxifen for,' he says, 'to stop it.' So I feel, from that, I feel the Tamoxifen isn't doing as well as it *might*.

Without the results of the scan and clear discussion with professionals, what might be called the 'limbo' of Bertha's suspicions remains intact. In fact, metastasis was suspected by the centre consultant at the time of the diagnosis of her recurrence, but not communicated to Bertha until several months later, when she was to return for palliative radiotherapy. Many patients enter into a veritable 'twilight zone' of ambiguous awareness when they enter the cancer illness calendar. The lack of dependable contact with an identifiable central treatment professional, or professional team, is a distinct feature of a confusing treatment context. Not knowing who is 'piloting the ship' as one patient put it, or who is in charge of what information, interferes with communication and relationship-building between professionals and patients.

'Key' professionals and helpers in the trajectory

'Key' professionals, or those seen as central to the treatment calendar (most usually those with high status, like consultants or surgeons), were assessed by patients in terms of their 'professionalism', including their management of the treatment calendar, and by their personal characteristics and manner. Professionals were discussed in interviews as professional *people*, not as mere 'figures' operating within rigidly defined roles. Professionals appeared in patients' accounts as narrative characters, whose thoughts, feelings and motivations were continually speculated upon.

A criterion of good treatment calendar management was 'open awareness', or the sensed possibility of it with key professionals. 'Approachability' was described as central to a more 'open' relationship. Betty, 44, a retired WREN with breast cancer, describes her surgeon in these terms:

> *BG:* Well it's the first time I've been in hospital since I was ten. As I say, I was quite impressed with his, patient–doctor approach, and that, if you had any questions you knew that you could, he would give you the answer, you know and, he wasn't morbid, he always had a smile on his face. He just had that, that manner, about him, he was so *very* approachable, you know you didn't think oh God, here he comes off the ward you know. Very, very relaxed but uh, you know he knows what he's talking about. You feel as though you're, that *he* knows what he's doing.

Feeling that the key treatment professional was a real 'person to talk to' as well as authoritative and direct was an acknowledged part of a good relationship with a key professional, as Jim, 63, a saw operator with cancer of the bladder, relates:

> *JW:* Well I thought Dr D was a bit more, like a person to *talk* to. I mean uh, Mr I [surgeon] he just pointed out what I . . . that's got to come out, so, typical Geordie you know. But uh, [Dr D] were really *nice* with you and all that you know, you could have a laugh with him. You knew where you stood with him and when he told you, 'That's it that's coming out and that's what's causing it they will have to come out, and I *want* you to come in', well, that sounds very clear to me.

On the other hand, feeling intimidated by a professional's 'manner' was discussed as a problem by many patients. A core aspect of a good personal manner was the presence of a 'personal touch' in dealings with patients. Its absence left 'professionalism' and technical skill intact, but appeared to ruin the chance for a real relationship (as characterized by trust, openness, and mutual exchange) to develop. Here Alice, 50, a business owner with breast cancer, describes an encounter with the radiotherapy consultant and his registrar:

> *AW:* . . . there was a feeling, oh I don't want to *go* there [the centre] any more and you know what I mean? *Got* to go, heh! But when, Dr D and that other lady doctor [senior registrar] came to see me, at [City B hospital], I found them much like sort of

scientists in their, I've *lost* the *word*. It really was all, it was like they'd, just walked straight out of a science lab . . . You know, they didn't seem to be there for very long. Dr L [registrar] said, 'The *main* thing is, do you have anything to ask?' As soon as she said it, in her *face*, I *knew* she must have a *horrible job* . . . she was so in*diff*erent, the conversation was only two minutes long, and I don't think the person . . . I *feel*, because Dr D was *not* very good at dealing with people he let *her* do it . . . I came out of that room not knowing *what* had been said, and *won*dered why the *heck* they'd come over to see me. I came away confused, disoriented and, just feeling I wished they hadn't bothered.

Alice here describes a potentially 'open' encounter (in which she is asked for her questions) being shut down through the manner of the professionals involved and the brevity of the consultation. In the interview from which this excerpt is taken, Alice was expressing fears that the radiotherapy consultant and registrar were keeping a more serious prognostic situation from her. In the above consultation, she was being told that several nodes had been affected by the cancer, and she would have to have extensive chemotherapy. She speculated at length about what this information 'really' meant, and whether she was being told she was terminally ill or not. In consultations with 'key' treatment professionals, patients are often being given information that is difficult to hear, and to interpret. Time, space and attention, all central treatment calendar resources in short supply in treatment settings, are central to such exchanges.

The apparent 'coldness' of the 'scientific' manner of these two key professionals is highlighted in this excerpt, but even with a warm professional manner, lack of *time* for discussions was also described as undermining to relationship-building with professionals. Here Adam, 58, a retired textile worker with lung cancer, describes the faultless 'professionalism' of his surgeon:

AL: I don't think that, from a *professionalism* . . . I don't think there is, I mean, they do their *job* and they do it *ex*cellent. But it's just that, margin of time, that you could do with that bit more. I mean, Mr M [surgeon] I mean he were, I've seen him on them wards seven o'clock on a morning, then back at nine o'clock at night, well, it's *de*votion isn't it? *Mar*vellous chap he is and then he's going back down to London as well. Calls his own patients [at outpatients' clinic] he does, nurse doesn't call them in. Being stood there waiting to shake hands with you at the door and that sort of thing . . . He's a smashing bloke.

Patients expressed admiration for the very busyness of the professionals they wished had more time for them, but the lack of a consistent relationship with one or more key professionals was cited as one of the most difficult aspects of treatment experience.

The test of a truly 'open' relationship with a key professional was whether or not difficult issues could be broached, including criticisms or questions about professional judgement. Maeve, 48, a housewife with breast cancer, describes 'gearing up' to have a confrontation with her surgeon over his mis-diagnosis of benign breast disease, resulting in a lengthy delay and several subsequent surgeries to remove a multi-focal breast cancer:

> MF: I've thought about it since you don't uhm, you don't start arguing with people when you first come for an operation. And, I mean a surgeon isn't somebody that you come . . . go in with all your guns blasting and . . . and play war with and if you . . . you're still in their hands. But, I do want to know more of the, *more* why, if he *knows* why, which, I don't know, seems kind of sad I feel . . . I just had the feeling that he was avoiding me. Or he felt guilty about the hospital thing I don't *know*. Maybe just me, but I will, I'll ask him.

Alice had also been misdiagnosed as having benign breast disease by her GP, who had not referred her for a mammogram when she had first con-sulted. She describes a relationship with her GP in which the difficult issue of initial misjudgement could be raised, post-diagnosis:

> AW: Well, he's only been in the practice about, *four* years I think, p'raps more, but I suppose it's just a *hu*man *na*ture thing that what you need is somebody that, you *feel* you can say, anything to. And I never went to see another doctor if *he* was available there*af*ter because, so many doctors think women are neurotic, and you feel guilty trying to tell them, trying to ex*plain* some-thing, and *don't* open up to them, because, *you* know, they feel women in general are neurotic. Soon as I met this one, I *could* talk to him. He *lis*tens, and he doesn't make you feel as though you're wasting his *time* which, *I* know I wouldn't dream of wasting a doctor's time, but *they* don't do they? I've even told him that I thought he should have sent me for a mammogram.

The possibility of such openness becomes more important over time, once the initial impact of diagnosis and early treatment has lessened, and the struggle to construct a meaningful context for events progresses. A consistent relationship with a key professional is increasingly important in the long-term context of cancer treatment and surveillance calendars. Amy, a 78-year-old housewife with lung cancer, describes the 'personal touch' of her connection with one of several key professionals in just such a context:

AE: *Ooh* Mr H, he's ever so good.
Husband: Oh he's an exceptional =
AE: = He puts his arm round me, he takes me down to see Dr D
            right from the basement to the . . . he walks me down to
            the basement he puts his arm round my shoulders all the
            way. And I don't ask for any special treatment I don't treat
            Mr H any different to how I treat anybody else but he
            always seems to, I don't know what it is, can't do enough
            sort of thing. Now, this has been going on for about five
            years, with Mr H.

The 'personal touch' and consistent contact over time seemed to increase
the value of relationships between patients and professionals.

Within the treatment calendar, professionals were heard, through patients'
accounts, to be presenting themselves to patients at times in specific, carefully managed ways. Dr D, the radiotherapy consultant at the treatment
centre, was praised highly for his approachability, informativeness and 'real
person' manner by male patients, while several women said they felt he
was not a 'good communicator' at all (see Alice's account, above). Bronwyn,
58, a catering assistant with cancer of the chortoid, describes an encounter
with Dr D during which she was told about the considerable effects of her
planned four-week radiotherapy treatment:

BG: Dr D was my hardest one, because he seems to, *pause* in
            between, *tell*ing you things. *I* nearly come to, get off that
            table, I *real*ly did, 'cause he *pau*ses. He *read*, these, ques-
            tions out and then he said, uh, 'Does it damage the brain
            cells?' [a question Bronwyn's husband had written out to
            be answered]. *Well*, and you see I thought *ooh*!
Husband: Every statement he made, he paused and, and he waited to
            see what the reaction was and it was like a body-blow you
            know 'cause I had, me arm round her, and I could feel her
            shrinking backwards every time he said something.
BG: I thought *ooh* I'm going to be like a dried-up old prune by
            the time! This is what were going through me *mind*, and
            then he said, but your hair *will* grow back, and then, that
            wasn't so bad. But then you see we came home, and we're
            thinking, oh a *hour's* radium, *that* sounds a *lot*, you know
            but, *since* then we, we got this book, they gave us a book,
            and we *read* it and got all, questions we wanted to know.
            So we went back and *saw* him, it was *so* different, by the
            time . . . I think I have to have about ten *min*utes' radium
            treatment . . .

Bronwyn had had to be convinced by her daughter to read the centre's
introductory booklet, from which she learned that her treatment would

not be for an hour at a time, as she had thought, but a mere ten minutes, with an hour needed for set-up. The rather theatrical manner in which the consultant had apparently dealt with Bronwyn (presumably as a way of impressing the seriousness of what was to come upon her) was not an uncommon feature of encounters with key professionals, particularly at sensitive moments in treatment, when difficult (to hear) information was to be relayed.

In general, lower status treatment professionals (nurses and radiographers) were described as more accessible. They were seen by patients more frequently, for longer periods of time and more consistently, and performed most of the actual work of treatment in the post-surgical treatment calendar. This work involves much physical 'handling' of patients, and the skill and care of 'helpers' in performing it was continually remarked upon by patients in interviews. Here May, 53, a catering assistant with floor-of-mouth cancer, describes another important aspect of the 'personal touch' in treatment:

> MS: It were just this bloke, what do they *call* his name? He's *very* nice because even me *hus*band noticed that he's the only *one, re*ally, that went out and got us off the couch. You have no, I've no *go* in me just yet with this shoulder, *all* this shoulder's left me now. And my husband noticed he said he's the only one *really* May, put his hands behind your head, and made sure you came up *stea*dy.

Being surrounded by support staff and students as well as several high-status professionals could also have a comforting aspect, as Bronwyn's husband notes:

> BG: There was about *five* under Mr N who I saw.
> Husband: But I think it's a teaching hospital because they all had a look, to see what you had you see. I think that it *help*ed actually because, it wasn't contained, within just *us*, it was out in the open and everybody, knew about it and uh, well you could talk freely.

The highly unusual form of cancer Bronwyn had, brought with it an intensive professional involvement. Patients having particularly complex (and 'newer') surgical procedures also described greater professional involvement (a greater number of professionals and more time) in the hospital than did those whose surgeries were more mundane.

The cheerful, brisk efficiency of 'helpers' or support staff at the centre was a feature of patients' accounts of treatment. While this 'pleasantness' made treatment more palatable, and enabled the treatment calendar (in its daily aspect) to run more smoothly, its effects were not always described in positive terms. Abby, 44, an ex-nurse with recurring breast cancer, describes the point at which her 'real' experience as a patient began, while on the simulator, being marked for treatment of a recurrence in her breast. In addition to being a five-year survivor of breast cancer, Abby had been a top-level NHS manager prior to her initial diagnosis, and was well known and greatly respected within the local authority for which she had worked:

> AW: I learned at a very early age in nursing, and even as a nurse, that *all* patients when you become a patient, the vulnerablity of that situation makes you deaf, dumb, blind, you know there's *so* much going on. Even when you *know* the system, and even though you *know* the place very well, put you in a pair of pyjamas and the *dy*namics are *so* different, they *really are* . . . That group of people [consultant and registrars at the centre], *great*, because, of who I was, the job I did before, I was treated as an intelligent human being who there was a good dynamic between. But when I went round to the simulator, there was a radiographer there, 'Oh *Mrs* W!' '*Miss* W.' 'Oh don't worry everyone gets Mrs here!' There was this tone of, 'Come along now', patronizing, speaking as though I was slightly deaf, slightly stupid, 'Just going to paint a little bit of this ink on you' and so on and on and on.

The difference between Abby's reception 'upstairs' with the consultant with whom she already had a professional relationship and 'downstairs' amongst the radiographers, is marked as her transition to disempowered 'patient':

> AW: . . . And *then*, the conversation that went on above my head between them, was so technical, I mean I hadn't got a clue because it was all about measurements, I could have been lying there petrified for all they knew. But then I thought, this is *in*teresting, because this is in fact the first time, I have been treated as a patient, of where they have no knowledge of me, so basically I am a *real* patient, to them. Because I've always had preferential treatment, even when I've been to a strange hospital because I'd written my name. The first five minutes I'm an ordinary patient. Then there'd be some little nurse reading my notes, eyes widening, 'Oh my God' on her lips *rush*ing off to Sister, Sister rushing over to me, '*Oh* so sorry you've been waiting', end of my experience as a patient. So this was really the first time.

Key 'helpers' cropped up in the early treatment calendar context as lower status professionals with 'insider' knowledge to help patients interpret or 'deal with' diagnosis and treatment experience. Bronwyn's husband describes a 'chance' meeting with a nurse who was also a cancer survivor:

Husband: Well they were very crafty at [City A hospital] because, as we arrived there was a big nurse on there, she was a lovely lass. And she says to Bronwyn, soon as we'd sat down, what are you in for? And of course Bronwyn told her and she says, well this time last year, *I* was in for the same thing, but on me throat. And they got on like a *house* afire *these* two. As I listened to them I realised what, 'cause she said she wasn't from the ward permanently, and I've wondered if they'd put her there to talk to Bronwyn to settle her down, 'cause the therapy was very very good. As I sat and thought about this and she was still talking, as she was leaving I says to her, you're very good at your job! I think it was therapy for Bronwyn you see, but it was for me too because I was *very* worried.

Amongst this group of patients, there had been no routine, formal provision of counselling, with the exception of one breast cancer patient who had been offered it. Helen, a housewife of 63, describes comprehensive informational and emotional support from the nurses on her hospital ward:

HB: The *first* time I just saw the *nur*ses, or radiographers. The second time, I think I saw the same radiographer, but I didn't really recognize her. And I saw Sister S. I'd seen her before when I went and had this, cystoscopy [for a kidney infection at time of diagnosis], and of course *that* was all in the air, and it [breast cancer diagnosis] just took over from the cystoscopy, which was fading into insignificance. And a *very* nice young staff nurse, a young man, suggested that the sister come up and have a word with me, she's just, down the corridor, you know and, he asked her to come along and she came and talked to me. *Very* nice, gave me *all* her time and uh, same with the staff nurses on the ward. If you were puzzled about anything they'd *drop* what they were doing and give you all their attention. They were *very* nice, anything that *puzz*led you or anything like that, even if there was something that *wasn't* puzzling you and that, they volunteered this information, very helpful, like this business with the pills [Tamoxifen side effects].

Professional sharing of attention and time emerged from the interviews as a central feature of good treatment calendar management. Attention to 'details' (such as Helen's reaction to Tamoxifen) and the provision of sufficient time to explore concerns and answer questions are central to the quality of care. Ellie said she had found the attention of a counsellor helpful as she went through diagnostic procedures and then surgery and release from the hospital:

ER: Well, I haven't really *ask*ed for all that much [information]. There
was the breast care counsellor at [City B hospital], *she* was there
the *first* time [routine mammogram] *and* the second, *and* the
morning that I went for the x-ray, and you know before the
operation *she* was there. Well she stood behind me all the time,
I was sat and she was stood behind me, and she was *great*, you
know. 'Cause, you know they said don't move, and then she said
to me, 'Mrs R,' she says, 'you are allowed to breathe,' she says,
'you're not *breath*ing.' I says, 'Well I move when I breathe', she
says, 'Well you are allowed to *breathe*, don't pass out on us!
Start breathing!' [Laughs] She was *very* good . . . she gave me her
card, she said, 'If there's anything . . .', 'cause you know, they say,
'Have you got any *quest*ions?' Well you, you're that stunned you,
you know I said, 'No, I don't think there is anything but, probably when I get home', and she said, 'Well *here*'s my card and if
there's *any*thing you want to know, if you want to ask *any*thing
about, just ring me, at this number.'

Ellie was the only patient to receive counselling from a formally appointed,
'in-house' counsellor, in the context first of pre-diagnosis routine screening,
through to discharge from hospital. 'Helpers in the trajectory' are those
most involved in the 'caring' work of the treatment calendar, as well as
those most likely to grapple with the practical difficulties, schedule gaps
and delays that so frequently plague treatment. Helpers also spent significant time just 'being with' patients at sensitive times.

Professionals' management of the treatment calendar

Liaison constitutes a major quantity of the work done by professionals in
managing the treatment calendar, and it is here significant problems can
arise. Much liaison between professionals, and between professionals and
patients, is achieved through the sending of letters. Letters were often the
source of surprise information or treatment calendar delays when they
were delivered to the wrong people (the patient instead of another professional in the treatment calendar, or the wrong GP in the practice); sent at
the wrong time (treatment cards arriving at the patient's home before a
statement of diagnosis had been made); addressed to somebody else; or
given inadequate postage. Letters were employed as a means of relaying
the diagnosis (being read aloud by the GP to the patient), and were seen as
a potential means by which professionals could evade the task of having to
face difficult interactions with patients (a feeling expressed in sardonic references to letter sending in several interviews). Letters were often depicted
as a distinct means of disengagement of agents from the treatment calendar

management task. There was much voiced confusion over whether or not letters were being sent to GPs, or between institutions, and as to what the formal procedures were for letter sending and other forms of liaison between professionals. Here Adam's wife speculates:

> Wife: I mean, do they still *send* reports to doctors?
> AL: But the only thing, that made *me* wonder is because I was actually referred to [a City A hospital] *by* the [local hospital] not by me own GP. Now I wondered, if the reports went to Dr W and not to me own GP.
> Wife: Well don't they ask you for who your GP was?
> AL: *Oh* yes it was all, he was *definitely* on me notes who me GP was yeah, yeah.

GPs were described as central allies in the treatment calendar, in cases where they were well known to patients. Liaison between the hospital consultant and the GP, for example, was often haphazard, and many patients voiced complaints about the apparent lack of a 'system'. Here Liam, 73, a retired dental technician with a recurrence of cancer of the larynx, and his wife discuss this problem:

> Wife: The only thing is, there doesn't seem to be any liaison with our GP and he gets cross, because they never let him know anything. He feels a bit *out* of it. I mean we've known him for what, over 30 years. He says it happens a lot, there's no feedback from the hospital *to* the GPs.
> LC: There's such a big delay, in letting *him* know, by the time . . . I mean this *last* time I don't think he knew anything *about* it.

When there was a lack of liaison, treatment mistakes could be made. Below, Alice describes receiving a double dose of oestrogen-blocking drugs, one from the GP (for a problem with heavy periods) and one from the hospital:

> AW: And *then* a silly thing happened was, when I came home from hospital they gave me a box of tablets and said I have to take them every day, a small box . . . and then I went to the doctor's the following Monday, and *he* gave me some, and on the *box* it was a different *name*, now when you're feeling ill and a little vague, you're not with it as much as you should be . . . I was *tak*ing one of each. Then, by the end of the small box from the hospital, I saw the name, I can't remember, was it, Tamoxifen? Tamoxifen, and it was the *same* tablet [as those the GP had prescribed] but a different *shape*, and so I was actually taking twice the *dose* . . .

Alice's GP eventually contacted the consultant and senior registrar at the centre to straighten out the confusion. When letters were addressed wrongly, mistakes could be more dramatic. Here Kevin, 60, an unemployed security officer, describes finding out about his 'other' cancer while consulting the GP for his floor-of-mouth cancer:

> KC: As a matter of *fact*, when I went to see my own *doctor* about *this* [floor-of-mouth cancer] it wasn't until *then* that I found I had a leu*kaem*ia, because one of the other doctors [in the practice] had done the initial tests, so the whole . . . the In*firm*ary were writing to this *oth*er doctor, and the letters were in my *file*, but, because they weren't addressed to *my* doctor he hadn't *read* them, so I never found out. I was just told it was an imbalance in the red and white blood vessels, that's all. And then I found out, a few weeks ago, and then this on top of it as well.

GPs were often a crucial resource in the treatment calendar in terms of their liaison work, explanation of technical information, and in sharing explicit information from consultants or surgeons ('key' professionals were often much more frank with the GP in letters than with the patient). When patients felt they did not have an ally in their GP, either because they had little pre-established connection with a practice, or because of feeling that the GP was unapproachable or disinterested, this lack seemed to reduce significantly their feelings of security and trust in the cancer illness calendar as a whole. Below Gerald and his wife describe being cheered by the wording of a letter to their GP from the radiotherapy consultant about Gerald's treatment for lung cancer:

> Wife: Our GP read out word for word a letter that Dr D had written to him, and he said, you know that, he knew with him being, it sounds a bit funny, a young man, and in very good health in every other way that, he was going to treat it as quickly as soon as possible, and uh, it was quite an optimistic letter.
>
> GW: And uh, what was his wording, monitor? Sort of, he was going to throw in quite a detailed monitoring of the situation, and it was going to be some intense treatment anyway, that's what they said.

GPs could also be instrumental in cutting through the 'red tape' of organizing hospital tests and appointments with specialists, and in getting the treatment calendar started quickly, as Kevin describes:

> KC: And him knowing that I was going to the In*firm*ary, the following Monday, for blood tests *any*way, instead of him making the appointment, he wrote a letter to the specialist I was going to

see, for him to sidetrack a bit of the red *tape*. I've a form of leukaemia, and I was going for a normal routine check-up on *that*, and I give the letter to the specialist who rang Dr D [radio-therapy consultant] up, and he saw me the same morning while I were there. We cut a lot of working time out.

Other peripheral professionals were occasionally able to achieve small but significant smoothings-of-the-way during testing and treatment planning. Gerald describes an episode of good 'surveillance schedule' management at the hospital:

> GW: Now Dr P [hospital consultant] *also* said I was going to have a CT scan, and they made me an appointment for Tuesday the following week. When I went there they said, 'Oh he's waiting for you.' Now that's the first time I've gone along and there's been somebody waiting for me, it was as*toun*ding. And it was the chap, who ran the CT at [City A hospital], Dr C, *su*per fellow. He did the scan and he says, 'Oh are you having any trouble with your left kidney? Any pain?' I said, 'No', he says, 'You've got a dilated kidney there. But,' he said, 'are you going to have a CT, scan?' I said, '*Yeah*, they sent me over', he said, 'I haven't got you on my list' =
>
> Wife: = Well a*gain*, one hand doesn't know what the other's *do*ing.
>
> GW: He says, *you* come and see me before you leave and I'll arrange for it. And it was on the *Tue*sday, and I was *scann*ed on the Thursday.

Fortuitous meetings with such 'peripheral' (to the cancer illness calendar) professionals played a significant role in 'getting things done' quickly and smoothly.

Through patients' accounts, treatment calendar management in practice emerges frequently as a lower order task, to be dealt with by lower status 'helpers' or by peripheral professionals (those in charge of surveillance schedules for example). Management of the treatment calendar from senior professionals is often 'patchy', without a formally acknowledged structure or system. If the patient is lucky, he or she has a communicative 'key' professional, and a supportive 'helper' or two at critical moments, good, thorough surgical aftercare and continuity between the referring hospital and the treatment centre, with rationales given for changes to treatment or the calendar, and clear information about follow-up procedures for all the treatment calendars. All too often, questions about the effects trajectories of treatments and the forms of the treatment and surveillance calendars, as well as about the meaning of tests and procedures, and changes of plan in these areas, go unaddressed by those professionals in whose hands the treatment calendar rests.

Note

1 Tamoxifen has been called the 'British wonder drug' because of the apparent lack of 'serious' side effects associated with it. A large national randomized trial was launched in April 1992 involving 15,000 women at risk for (but not ill with) breast cancer to determine the success of the drug in preventing the disease in well women at risk. Doubt over the ethics of the trial and the safety of the drug (to be administered to the experimental group daily for five years) was expressed in both the popular and the academic presses ('Specialist rejects cancer drug health fears', *Guardian*, 5 March 1992; 'A question of prevention', *Guardian*, 6 March 1992; 'Trials and tribulations', *Guardian*, 4 August 1992; Letters, *Lancet*, 339, 15 February 1992). This debate points up the issue, among others, of 'side effects' and their definition: patients found it difficult to report 'symptoms' or problems to their treatment calendar managers that they had not heard as possibilities in descriptions of treatment at the outset. This underscores the importance of knowledge of the likely effects trajectory for patients and also for clinicians, who need to develop clinical pictures of treatments and their effects to improve medicines and practice.

Being treated: navigating the treatment calendar

In the previous chapter, our focus was on preparations for the start of the treatment calendar. The main elements of the treatment calendar at this stage were the lack of choice patients have over treatment; the impact of surgery; attempts to prepare for life in treatment; dealing with the losses caused by surgery; and the location of the various professionals in the treatment context. In this chapter we move to the actual experience of treatment and the work of the treatment calendar once it is properly under way. It must be remembered that 'the treatment calendar' for each patient will often be several discrete calendars run at the same time, some (like chemotherapy) lasting for a longer period of time than others. We will examine several main modes of treatment through patients' accounts of being treated. For the patient, the work of the treatment calendar involves interpreting its logic, and the meaning of changes within it. The time- and energy-consuming processes of going for treatment, dealing with its effects, attending reviews, and having to manage several modes of treatment (and several calendars) at the same time are major aspects of the experience of treatment that impact directly on patients' quality of life. The work of professionals in the treatment context has a direct bearing on how these quality of life concerns are dealt with.

The treatment work of the treatment calendar

The start of the treatment calendar brought about a change in the medical contexts of the illness experience for the patients interviewed here. The time of the treatment calendar was a time of greater simplification of the illness calendar for most patients, because a concrete plan was in place, involving one central institution and fewer key professionals. All those in the group were receiving radiotherapy at the treatment centre in City A. Three women were also having chemotherapy at the large referring hospital in City B and at the centre, both during and following their radiotherapy calendars. Two women with breast cancer had implanted wire treatment at the centre. In addition to these main modes of treatment, there was treatment to deal with 'side' effects (medications, creams and dressings, gastric feeding) and 'surveillance schedules' (Corbin and Strauss 1988) involving x-rays, CT scans, blood taking and regular radiotherapy reviews. For some patients, treatment meant becoming an in-patient, either for a special procedure (implanted wire treatment) or because the effects of treatment needed intensive medical management (dehydration and malnutrition with inability to swallow for one larynx and one floor-of-mouth cancer patient, for example). There was continuity at this stage in treatment, because the bulk of activity in the illness calendar was largely limited to one institution, the centre, one consultant, and (mostly) one registrar.

One major resources condition affecting the treatment calendars of all the patients interviewed at this time was the difficulty the centre was having with its overburdened radiotherapy machines. There had been several serious maintenance problems (ageing equipment pushed to capacity, unavailability of replacement parts from Europe, and difficulty getting the technical expertise to do repairs and maintenance), compounded by a large and expanding patient load. With two machines out of action or running at reduced capacity much of the time, there was a reduction of new patient uptake, which had created a backlog which then had to be cleared.

Radiotherapy

Liam, 73, a retired dental technician whose work had once involved him in making radiotherapy masks, describes the experience of radiotherapy treatment:

> LC: I can imagine it being frightening to some people. The very fact that, you're laid on a bed, and the mask comes down and is fastened onto the bed, you can't move, and then, this *great* big machine whirrs round. Then they *go, leave* you to it, and, *clatters* down this machine . . . oh it makes a terrible noise, a right *crack*. I used to count it 73 seconds in my own counting, I knew when it was coming, this big crack you see, but for anyone not *know*ing it . . . it might be a bit frightening. You see, they've nobody in the room – obviously they're monitoring it you see – they tell you, *if* at any time you want any help, just shout or something, we'll be here . . . But maybe there are people who would be scared . . . you're in this great big room, all by yourself,

nobody in there holding your hand. With your first two or three treatments they tell you what's going to happen and that, then after *that* it's just a question of *lay* still, fasten you down, you lay there and then, slip out, slip in again and change it round, and then when you hear little footsteps coming you know it's finished you see.

Maggie, 50, a housewife with breast cancer, describes the rather hi-tech and immaculate nature of radiotherapy:

MG: I *won*dered what, what – how – what – how, it was *like*, I'd never ever seen anything before, any mach*ine* of any kind but I suppose you just feel as though you're on an operating table [laughs] with a machine above you up there, lined up next to the part that has to be treated, and then they just seem to switch something on and there's just like a zzz, a buzzing noise you can't actually *feel* anything *then*, you know and then uhmmm, that's it, everybody's programmed [sighs] I *think*, for as limited a time as you have to have, you know I think they run a *tape* out there someone, someone said a tape, push a tape in and it's recorded like, and uh, you're on a machine.

Many patients described monitoring treatment themselves by counting the seconds the 'buzzing' noise lasted for each field. Adam, 58, a retired textile worker with lung cancer, describes asking why treatment appeared to last longer at times:

AL: One question I *did* ask I couldn't understand when I were on treatment they set you up for the first field of course which was a *front* and, when they go out of the room, you can hear it come on it, you know it starts *buzz*ing, can't feel or see anything but it used to have . . . I got in the habit of *coun*ting, to see how long it was you see. Anyway what I'd had three or four treatments over four days and, I says to 'em, 'Have you in*creas*ed my amount of treatment I'm having in each field?' and they says, 'No *why?*' So I tell them I counted how many times, you know, I get to 30 or so, and it'd go off, next minute I'll get to 50 or 60, and it'd go off. 'Oh,' she says, 'We don't *set* it for *time*, we, set it for the amount of power you *want* but if, other machines are working at the same *time*, it takes *longer* to give that,' – which were worth *ask*ing really 'cause I thought it were very strange. I mean I thought if, it's you're counting fast or, you're not counting as fast as you did yesterday and *that* sort of thing.

As Adam explained, 'radiation is a killer really, isn't it?', and patients expressed a concern to know that they would not be overexposed. It took time in treatment before patients asked questions about the detail of how radiotherapy worked and was managed. Abby, 46, a retired nurse and NHS manager, describes asking finally a question about what had been bothering her since treatment set-up:

> AW: It's the same sort of thing, you know, the doctor comes along and says, 'OK Mrs Bloggs, I'm going to cut off your head and graft on a cabbage', 'Oh thank you doctor!', you know, take it *all* and never question. Not question because you think they're *wrong*, but more, 'What's this about', you know, 'You're going to do this to me' . . . I thought, if I've got rays coming here, here, here and *here*, *how* come it's not destroying every chopping bit of tissue that's between all of that? You know, a bit of heart, a piece of lung, an ascending aorta! Which I thought was a very sensible question and apparently yes it *was* a very sensible question. And she said, 'No one's ever asked us that before.' I mean I *know* enough to ask.

Learning about the degree of precision involved in targeting the radiation so as to prevent or reduce damage to healthy tissue was described as comforting to patients who, in the absence of side effects early in their schedules, wished to know what the radiation was doing inside their bodies. Effects did surface as time went along, often with a vengeance. Liam, a veteran of radiotherapy, having been treated with it extensively for a first diagnosis of larynx cancer 15 years before his recurrence, describes the effects trajectory of radiotherapy for head and neck cancer patients like himself:

> LC: A fortnight after I started, the pain began, which is when it takes effect, and it lasts . . . it lasts a fortnight after you've finished. You see, you've got the radiation *in* you evidently, or so it's been explained to me, by the nurses, and it takes effect . . . you don't sort of come home and say, 'Oh now I've finished treatment. I'm all right.' Because, my throat here was *black*. The skin was black and it was all peeling. *Really* burned. Well that, gradually got *worse*, even after I'd finished treatment. You can say it's a fortnight after you start to a fortnight after you finish. The first fortnight you don't feel any effect at all.

Patients with head and neck and lung cancers were those reporting the most severe effects (severity seemed contingent on individuals' tissue strength and general well-being going into treatment, age and so forth), while breast cancer patients described feeling little different from normal as they went through treatment, though skin became darker (as with a deep tan) and sometimes red and sore towards the finish of the schedule, and a pervasive tiredness became a problem around the middle to after the finish of schedules. Abby's treatment was more extensive than that of the other breast cancer patients interviewed, as her recurrence of multi-focal breast cancer was diffuse and hard to target. She describes the enervation that can be a significant effect of radiotherapy for many patients:

> AW: After my first week in treatment, I was in Sainsbury's one evening and my first spasm of, 'Oh my God my legs won't move!' *hit* me. It was like hitting a wall, for an hour or so. My legs turned to jelly, I thought God I feel tired. And it was just like with chemo, only with chemo it lasts longer.

Bronwyn, a housewife of 58, was being treated to her head for a cancer that had started at the back of her (now removed) left eye. Bronwyn's treatment involved an hour of set-up for several fields, so with the two hours' driving time to the centre from her village, in addition to the waiting time at the centre and the treatment time, 'treatment' could mean a full day each weekday, from 8.30 in the morning until 3.00 in the afternoon. Her husband, a merchant seaman, drove her to treatment daily:

> BG: I used to come off that machine and, come back through we used to go for this cup of tea now it weren't so bad, but by the time I got home I was *jiggered*, you know, so it's that *journey* isn't it . . . I don't know how these poor people go on what are going on ambulances though and have to go *around* and about but . . . it's one way of getting there isn't it?

While the 'side' effects of radiotherapy could be severe (especially for head and neck and lung patients, requiring hospitalization for some people and gastric feeding), the rigours of the outpatient radiotherapy treatment calendar added to the total effect of treatment on each individual. Being a patient in treatment for cancer was a full-time job.

Implanted wire treatment

In addition to four-week radiotherapy schedules, two women had implanted wire treatment. This involved an in-patient stay in an isolated ward (with telephone, television and toilet facilities) for three to five days, with visitors, including staff, restricted to ten- to fifteen-minute stays. In this type of treatment, radioactive wires are inserted into rods implanted in the breast with the patient under a local anaesthetic. Ellie, a retired catering assistant of 64, describes the procedure:

> ER: When I came back from the operating theatre there was seven, like very fine *rods*, they put through, and then, the doctor *came*

with this canister, like this, I opened it up and saw these, well they looked like, fine plastic wires, but like white, things stuck out. And he just tucked *one* and slid it inside these tube . . . these rods and then, he cut it off, to the length he wanted, then put like this metal stuff along and fastened it with a *screw*driver [laughs] . . . it *did*n't hurt or anything though just, so I didn't, look. And that's what they did with all of the seven, they just kind of put the, and at *this* side there was little rubber stoppers, you know to stop the wires sticking in you I s'pose. And they just tightened each one up and that so's it was lined up . . . they went in at *that* side and came out at that side.

The worst aspect of the treatment was apparently the way it looked ('gruesome') under the bandage and when being removed, and the isolation from family and friends:

ER: I kept thinking about all these *hos*tages you know, I mean they've been out all these years! And I kept thinking I've only been here four days and yeah, I think it's just that, just a lack of company really, you're just on your own all the time.

Rachael, a supply teacher of 41, describes feeling anxious and 'jumpy' during her stay, though she was not sure why:

RS: I wasn't *frigh*tened, I had *plen*ty to do and people kept *ring*ing me, and it was annoying me in a way when they rang me because I mean oh I've got to stand *still* and *lis*ten to you while you talk to me and I . . . I felt *jum*py and I don't know *why*, it didn't *hurt* particularly it was, it were discomforting but, maybe my *body* was frightened I don't know.

Ellie described the most difficulty with the removal of her wires, and with staff protocol regarding who was allowed to enter the room and for how long:

ER: It's heavy stuff you know it's all, radiation. Actually he [doctor removing rods] wasn't too pleased when he took all the seven out to*geth*er. He couldn't get them *in*to this *box*, and the lid down, so he had to take each one out of this, bar and drop it in and then drop the bar and put the lid down and he said to the lady who was with him, that he weren't too pleased about that 'cause he said the three of us had been exposed to these rods, longer than we *need*ed to be. I think he wanted a bigger box next time, but I don't know if this is a new treatment or *not* because, you'd have thought they'd, already worked that *out* that, *that* wouldn't go into that box.

Knowledge of protocol for the management of patients with this type of treatment seemed a problem for the support staff at the centre:

> *ER:* You see a lot of the staff . . . not the *nurs*ing staff but a lot of the auxiliaries, they didn't seem to understand whether they could come in or not. One lady with iodine treatment had to have her own *cup*, saucer, all her own – *they* kept coming and says, 'Do you,' you know, 'is that *your* cup or can I take it away?' I says to one of the nurses, 'It's a pity somebody doesn't explain to these auxiliaries what it's all about', she says, 'We *do*' [laughs], as if . . . we *do*, quite often, so I said, 'Oh dear, it's like that is it!'

The handling of the hazardous substances involved in cancer treatment (including chemotherapy) seemed problematic at times in the treatment calendar. As early as two years prior to Ellie's and Rachael's experiences, interstitial wire treatment had been given on ordinary wards, behind lead screens. A greater respect for the hazards of this treatment seemed to have informed its administration since, though not without hitch.

Chemotherapy

Chemotherapy was performed on an outpatient basis both at the treatment centre in City A and the referring hospital in City B. At the centre, either the radiotherapy consultant's senior registrar gave the treatment, or it was administered by a specialist nurse, in a special chemotherapy ward. There was no such provision at the City B hospital, with chemotherapy sometimes given by centre staff at special outpatient clinics there, and at other times by hospital nurses and registrars with no special training in administering chemotherapy (the lack of trained in-house staff at the hospital in City B was a contentious issue for centre consultants, who wanted to see a special ward set up at the hospital to accommodate City B chemotherapy patients). The lack of a regular 'set-up' for chemo treatment at City B hospital caused problems for several patients, as Melissa, 49, a university housekeeper with breast cancer, and her husband describe:

> *Husband:* Once again, last time we went for chemotherapy at [City B hospital] we found out that was, uhm an*xiety*, wife was, it was a *hell* of a long wait wasn't it when you were there last time. Did you go there =
> *MG:* = Half-past one, it was quarter past *four* . . .
> *Husband:* It was quarter past four the time we went in which, for anybody suffering, like such as like, with pains or something like that, is a long time to wait. But I mean that was explained to us that only one person come through from

[City A treatment centre] and, this, they were giving the treatments and this is why, it was so I mean obviously you accept it but when you're sat there you know you're stuck in waiting room for three hours or, two and a half hours it seems an eternity though.

Here Betty, 44, a retired WREN with breast cancer, describes the difference in receiving treatment in the two places:

BG: The first time [at City B hospital] it was basically, compared to the second time, just shoved in if you get my drift, I mean *I* wouldn't know how it was going to be administered, you know straight into the *arm*, *one* thing after another, you know, ten minutes right, you go *home* now ... The *sec*ond time I was administered through at [the centre] on the *ward* and that was administered by a nursing sister, two nursing sisters, and it *seem*ed that the *whole* atmosphere was so relaxed I mean it was all [that particular ward] was obviously *for*, the giving of chemotherapy you know. Nice easy armchair, with a pillow and that. They had problems trying to find a vein in my arms [laughs slightly] you know. That was administered completely *diff*erently, that was, it was in my *hand*.

Treatment sessions lasted about 15 minutes, with a blood test first to see if the blood count was high enough to permit treatment. The impact of each treatment tended to differ widely from session to session and woman to woman. Generally, reactions were not of a 'crisis' nature (although Melissa had uncontrollable vomiting the day after her third treatment and needed treatment from her GP), with enervation and nausea common. The women experienced some hair thinning (though not alopecia), fevers and rashes that tended to be short-lived. The biggest problem tended to be a deep and pervasive fatigue that suddenly descended at points during the day and made it difficult to pursue or plan personal calendar activities. Betty describes being surprised at how well she felt during her chemotherapy calendar, compared with what she'd feared it might be like:

BG: Because, of the *two* [modes of treatment: radiotherapy and chemotherapy] the *word* chemotherapy you know, throwing up in the toilet bowl all the time and your hair's falling out and this that and the other, of the *two* that was the one I feared most, about the symptoms. But then of course there was these other women and some of these women would come in the morning looking *aw*ful, and I'd be in there bright as a button you know ... I felt quite good about that you know, after about three or four days, after the initial shock had subsided it's not been actually bad, hasn't been that bad.

The impact of the chemotherapy was worsened by radiotherapy treatment and the process of travelling to the centre from a distance away for treatment, as Alice, 50, a business owner with breast cancer relates:

AW: The first time I was left sat in, sitting in a *chair*, and I just didn't know where to put me body, and the girl that had done the chemo went off *du*ty, and, because of this dreadful tiredness you're just *half*-cooked. I just *sat* there and I didn't *say* anything to anybody and I *should* have said, 'Do you mind if I lie down? I'm not well.' They asked me later how I'd felt and they said, 'We'll make a note of it.' Now the *following* time I'd been out of the house, ever so many hours by the time I'd had the chemotherapy that, rather than me *stay* another two hours, they'd got the ambulance to hang on so that I could come back home, and we'd *everybody* to drop off, and the time I was in the *am*bulance I just didn't know where to put me body.

As indicated here, the rigours of the treatment calendar itself contribute a great deal to the impact of treatment substances, even given smooth administration. Small details of treatment administration (like whether one is asked how one feels afterwards, and whether the treatment professional remains at hand) are likely to be important to 'handling' it well. In addition to chemotherapy and radiotherapy effects, and travel back and forth for treatment, the women had all had lumpectomy and lymph node removal with lingering effects from the surgery. It remained unclear as to the extent to which the various modes interacted to produce certain effects, and what would happen after each successive treatment. Alice found the effects lessened after her third chemotherapy treatment, while Melissa had a violent reaction to her third for the first time. She described feeling concerned that she was 'getting worse' and was puzzled, 'after I'd done so well with me radiotherapy'. The continued challenges of interpreting the effects of treatment was a major task in managing life in the treatment calendar for these women.

Treatment calendar consistency, alteration and change

Patients described monitoring treatment closely, and were concerned about the amount of radiation to which they were being exposed. They wondered aloud about how their schedules compared with those of other patients, and what the significance was of the number of fields treated. Adam, 58, a retired textile worker with lung cancer, expressed the concern that he might be having three times the treatment that he was initially prescribed:

AL: When I went for me treatment I had no idea that I were going to have three phases. You know p'raps they could have explained, you know that I were going to have it in three different places, I was under the impression you know I'd go and they'd just slap it onto a place and that'd be it. I mean *I* feel I don't know whether it *is* so that, you're having three times the volume of anybody that's only having say one phase or two phases. I don't know whether that's correct or not. Or whether the volume is split into the three fields.

The reasoning behind a particular schedule, and the significance for the underlying question, 'How ill am I?' of treatment detail, was reportedly rarely addressed during the radiotherapy schedule, although patients described getting some technical questions answered by radiotherapy staff, as Gerald, 67, a retired engineer with lung cancer describes:

GW: I was asking in the finish, *why* they had done one, done it *one* way and then another. Because they did me ten treatments through here and through the back, the machine came right the way round, 360 degrees, and then the next ten, there was one down there and then two in from the side so I was just asking this lad on the last day and he says, 'Well *ac*tually what we did in*iti*ally we were *shrink*ing the tumour, and then we were attacking it.'

Understanding the rationale behind treatment calendar changes, whether pre-planned or not, was central to understanding treatment as a rational process, with sometimes several goals and aims.

Daily inconsistencies in the radiotherapy calendar resulted from machine breakdowns and from the unpredictable juggling of different types of patients (self-transport, ambulance and in-patient), as well as the unique doses, positions, numbers of fields treated and so forth that form each person's prescribed daily treatment. As two patients pointed out, one's time in treatment each day depended partially on the nature of *other* patients' treatments beforehand. In managing daily inconsistency, patients described feeling 'in the dark' as to the reasons for delays. At the outset, little was understood about the implicit protocol of the clinic. As time went on, patients became more aware of the reasons for delays and changes to the schedule, although these tended not to be explained directly. They often 'found out the hard way', as Ellie, 64, a retired catering assistant with breast cancer, describes:

ER: What happened that *day*, was when we got there, the ma*chine*s broke down, they got going a*gain* but there was this, there was somebody in front of me and then me and then this lady opposite, and then two *more* came in. Well, *these* two the nurses said will you come *this* way, and they'll take you to the other machine,

so *they* went you see. And *this* person went that *was* in front of
me, and then they come for this other lady. And I said *oh* it's *my*
turn 'cause I'd been sat there about an hour. And so, this nurse
said oh I'm *sorry* but she didn't say *why*, this lady has to go so
she *went*, so, I says to Mrs S [another patient] I said I'm *sorry* I
didn't mean to be, it's me before you sort of thing but, anyway
my appointment *was* before hers. But *afterwards* I found out that
the reason *why*, was they didn't want to alter the setting – it
takes quite a bit to get the machines set. And hers was . . . *this*
other man must have been for his throat you see and hers was
too so. But they didn't tell me that you see, so I didn't really
understand it.

Not knowing how long a treatment day was going to be caused strain for
many people. Ambulance patients could never be quite sure that the ambulance would turn up at pre-set times, and planning the day was difficult, as
Bertha, 62, a retired clerk with metastatic breast cancer, describes:

BB: I was very slightly sick . . . Well actually what happened was me
appointment was 1.30, now the ambulance picked me up here, I
was told to be ready for 12.30. Well it got here at 11.45, which
finally got to [City A centre] at half past *two*! So, the ambulance
to bring me home came over to me and another lady that were
having treatment, and they were actually waiting for me, before
I had me treatment on the shoulder. So of course I was sort of
straight out of the treatment into the ambulance, and I was just
feeling a bit nauseous by the time we came. And uh I came in, all
I'd had was a slice of toast since six o'clock!

Many patients' spouses and other family members accompanied them to
treatment, and for these people, treatment was a shared experience. Delays
could be a source of worry to family members who 'lost track' temporarily
of patients who were delayed in treatment. Terry's wife became worried
about her husband when he was delayed in the treatment room. He had
been left strapped to the treatment table while the radiologists left the room,
and the machine had malfunctioned. Because Terry had a heart condition,
his wife feared he had had a heart attack when he failed to reappear at the
usual time:

Wife: That's another thing – the flaming machine broke down didn't
it when we were in on the Monday, and uh, the radiologist
didn't know 'cause she was out of the room. I were worried
stiff 'cause I thought he's in a long *time* you know and it had
broken down the computer wasn't working or something just
. . . they didn't take it off [Terry's treatment mask] until they'd
had a break you know, just carried on with the treatment.

The suspended animation of waiting to be called in to treatment, but never quite knowing when, was described by many people, patients and spouses alike, as one of the hardest aspects of the daily experience of radiotherapy. Waiting exerted a 'low-level stress', as one person put it, that wore people down. Helen, 63, a housewife with breast cancer, describes this type of stressful situation:

> HB: The *worst* thing has been the sitting around and waiting for a turn. *Sure*ly that wasn't necessary. And you get the *feel*ing that if you're, it's a bit old-fashioned, it goes back to the old days when you just sat there and you ex*pect*ed to sit there for hours ... and *al*so, on top of that, no explanation as to *why* you're not, or how long you're going to be, you *go* on and then, and they say I'm sorry you have to wait. Sometimes it comes over the grapevine that, the machine's broken or something happened. Just, being *left* there, and then, you go for your turn and that's it and you're home. That in a way is a little bit of an, anti-climax? ... You get taken in a different order sometimes so you're just in the dark until your *name* is called. And then it's all over, straight away, and you're *out*, and *that*'s quite stressful.

Travelling to and waiting for treatment are major aspects of the radiotherapy treatment calendar that complicate the impact of radiotherapy itself. Ambulance patients in particular had considerable time added to their daily treatment calendar, as described by Dan, 76, a retired quantities surveyor with urinary tract cancer, explaining why he had decided to 'give in' and become an in-patient for a week towards the end of his treatment calendar:

> DG: But *Oh* I'd had enough, I just couldn't take any more. I'd had the four weeks, four weeks of it. I was into the fifth *week* because of holidays and machines breaking down, but I'd had four weeks of travelling to [City A] every day, and believe me there's no pleasure in travelling in the ambulances or, *terr*ible ...
> KC: Worse than the bus?
> DG: O*OOh what*! [laughs] At least we would have been comfortable on a bus but our knees every time you went over a *peb*ble, you know, the whole uh, machine juggered you know it just wasn't one, piece, oh no it was most uncomfortable.

A lengthened treatment calendar due to resources problems and general calendar events (bank holidays) is made more difficult for Dan by the rigours of ambulance travel. The transport ambulances required patients to sit loosely strapped onto seats along the sides of the vehicle, twisting and turning along city streets stopping at homes and institutions to collect people for treatment each day. Patients with their own transport voiced concerns about their ability to drive themselves back and forth. All patients but one came with a companion, a neighbour, friend or spouse, in case of problems. Neighbours and friends worked out rosters for this work. Patients packed tonics, anti-nausea tablets and plastic containers in case they became sick on the way home.

Daily inconsistency was a fact of life in treatment. Structural change in the treatment calendar invariably meant that the calendar was lengthened as well as qualitatively changed for many patients. Change to the treatment calendar was experienced by all the patients in the form of a lengthened calendar owing to machine breakdowns, backlogs and bank holidays. The prescription of a supplementary, 'booster' schedule added extra time for many (the fact that scans were being taken for the booster set-up and not for some other purpose was not routinely explained to patients). Problems like these often combined to become more major delays, as Terry describes here:

> *TL:* The last treatment, it would've worked out that . . . on the Friday was the other machine's maintenance day, uh, on *each* of the machines [in Terry's treatment calendar] so instead of . . . I had to go every day just the same but only got, one treatment on one machine *one* day and one machine the following day so I lost one day out of it. That meant, instead of having the final treatment on the Friday, it was the following *Mon*day, the Monday was a bank holiday and so was Tuesday, so the *final* treatment I'd to wait four *days* in effect to finally get along with it. And then when I went to the final treatment, I was feeling better for my four days off, and then she said it was *so* bad she didn't want to treat it!

The radical radiotherapy calendar for most patients was actually comprised of two schedules, the initial fractions and the 'booster' schedule. However, the treatment card handed to patients at prescription described only the initial schedule. While patients were generally told the approximate length of the total calendar, they assumed that the number of fractions on their appointment cards was the total number of treatments. This caused distress to those who suddenly 'discovered' they were to have further treatment. May, 53, a pub caterer with floor-of-mouth cancer, had been trying to conceal her considerable side effects from the radiographers in order to escape being made an in-patient, thinking she was nearing the end of the treatment calendar. She was admitted as an in-patient at the insistence of radiographers, with malnutrition and dehydration, and an additional nine treatments ahead of her:

MG: *They* told me wrong. It were on me card eleven treatments see, and when it comes out it *was*n't eleven, it were eleven and nine . . . if I'd have done the Friday's, I'd have got me eleven *done* with. And so I didn't want to *say* anything about me not eating and swallowing you see, I wanted to come home and go there and then I would have it *done* with. And then it were a nurse that's in radio— where machines are themselves. She said, 'How are you coping?' I said, 'Well I'm not' – but I didn't know what I were doing then telling *them* you see but they shot up at doctor straight a*way*, they made me stop there while I got on we got a bed. I said, 'Well, can't I come home and come back and stop in tomorrow? And then I've got me eleven done with', and *that's* when they've, brought bombshell on me, you've, how many more of them left? It were up to *twen*ty.

May had had to recuperate for two weeks before resuming another three weeks of treatment as an in-patient, totalling five weeks of hospitalization. More explicit knowledge of the treatment calendar at outset might have prevented her from obscuring her deteriorating condition from staff until she was over halfway through her calendar. Had her eating and fluid intake been addressed earlier, some of her hospital stay (which was at outset, essentially 'crisis management') might not have been necessary. Patients' lack of knowledge of their treatment calendars can interfere with *their* treatment management and with their communication with professionals, and result in a drain on clinic resources.

Some chemotherapy patients had their treatment calendars extended as they were nearing the completion of the calendar. They had not been told of this possibility, and described the change as demoralizing. The addition of a single extra chemotherapy treatment meant that, in effect, the treatment calendar was extended for three weeks, as there was a three-week break between sessions during which side effects had to be dealt with. Each treatment session brings unpredictable effects and an indeterminate period for recovery, complicating a return to full participation in the personal calendar. Here Betty, 44, a retired WREN with breast cancer, describes the implications of structural change:

BG: I mean when they say, 'Oh well we'll give you three months, then I'm prepared to . . .', you know. So you go home when you know the intervals you can work it out. So, January the 10th is a free month [finish of chemotherapy schedule]. All right, we'll give you an *ex*tra one. It'll make me sick so, you add another 21 days.

Within this uncertain trajectory is the underlying issue of what *therapeutic* effect the treatment is having, something the patient may not find out for some time ('We'll give you three months, then I'm prepared to . . .').

Professionals' work in the treatment calendar

It has been argued that the modern physician is distinguished by his or her function as the *manager* and not solely as the *provider* of treatment (Arney and Bergen 1984), and a prominent theme in the 1990s debates about health care management is the image of clinicians as the managers of resources (Elston 1991), despite the barriers created by an NHS culture and thus environment geared to administration rather than management (Cox 1991). The chief resource considered in this discussion of the management work of the treatment calendar, and of its impact on the personal calendar, is that of *time*. Time is precious to both patients and professionals; it is in short supply for patients who find that treatment has taken over their daily lives, and for professionals who must distribute and ration their time (and thus their expertise) so as to perform the work of treatment. For patients, the threat to the resource of time posed by a cancer diagnosis is literally a matter of life and death. For professionals, the stakes are lower, and time management is restricted to management of professional *work* within time constraints. This is an important distinction, and one that creates a subtle but pervasive tension in the treatment situation. It is through recognition of this contextual feature of treatment that the full significance (for the patient) of the treatment calendar professional as treatment calendar *manager* emerges.

Lower status staff and the work of treatment and schedule management

The 'nitty gritty' of the daily treatment schedule (treatment itself, monitoring, aftercare, daily clinic and individuals' schedule management) was the province of nurses, radiotherapy technicians and aides, and ambulance staff at the treatment centre. Several patients saw the dietitian, and one patient had physiotherapy at the centre. Patients praised centre staff for the 'tone' of the centre which they described as 'upbeat', and as a product of the pleasantness and efficiency of the staff. Derek, 60, a taxi driver with larynx cancer, describes the 'ordinariness' of the rhythm of treatment:

> DM: They you know, they're very nice. They... they make you feel you're not poorly, it's all, it's just, well not a *game* I mean it's definitely not a game it's just, an ordinary day thing you know, I...I haven't felt it hasn't made me feel more poorly, it hasn't done that. You know it's like going to the supermarket, they make, they make it so easy. They have, they've made it very easy.

Consistency in the treatment calendar was achieved in the contact patients and family members had with the same staff members each day. Here Sam,

63, a building contractor with melanoma, describes the feeling of personal attention generated by consistent contact:

> SM: We, we *all* agree I think that the staff up there are very good, at [the centre]. I've experienced hospital staff since I've been to [the centre] and I think they're, they're a little bit more caring at [the centre] . . . You can see a look in their eyes like, well although you're on computer, they don't have to use it, and that is nice, and I think it, *makes* you feel nice, and it puts you at ease.

Apart from overseeing and running the daily schedule of the waiting room, staff were responsible for monitoring each patient's progress with regards to 'side' effects and general condition. This involved eliciting information from patients, as well as answering their questions. This was accomplished with persistence and subtlety by radiographers who always 'got what they wanted' out of patients, as Terry and his wife describe:

> *Wife:* They have a way of prising out what you do as well haven't they?
> TL: Well they would say, 'Are you managing to, can you still swallow?', you know, and I'd say, 'Yes', 'Well what . . . what did you have *yester*day?', sort of thing you know . . .
> *Wife:* You know, chicken soup, *oh*. They have a crafty way of getting . . . I thought they were very nice.

Part of the work of treatment for staff involved detailed monitoring of how patients were coping with the side effects of treatment, interpreting and treating new physical problems that appeared, and making referrals to the consultant. Bronwyn, 58, a catering assistant with cancer of the chortoid, describes this work as a feature of the daily process of going for treatment:

> BG: Them *girls* are very helpful because, when I was having all these *pains* you know they were, they was concerned about it. And, one of the girls said, 'Well have you had a new *limb* or anything?' So I said well *yes* I had, so she said, 'Well we better have *that* made out to, to doctor', you see. That's how, they know I had this trapped . . . it was on a trapped *nerve*, 'cause it [eye prosthesis] wasn't made *larg*er. . . You see, as they come for you they'll . . . the *first* day they asked you, who you are your name, address and telephone number and everything. But *af*ter that, they just say, 'Come along Bronwyn', you know, and, ever so *friend*ly. And then they would say, 'Now then how are you?' This is all walking to, that room, and you had to tell them what you thought and that and, if *they* thought you should see doctor well you went to see the doctor and, that way.

Radiography and nursing staff were instrumental in helping to interpret the effects of treatment for patients, offering understandable explanations, as Liam, 73, a retired dental technician with throat cancer, recounts:

LC: I mentioned it to the nurses there, and I said, 'Well it's feeling a bit rough.' They said, 'Well don't forget, it's *peel*ing there, imagine if the inside of your throat's like *that*! It starts like that, and it's going to get worse you see!' But oh, they were smashing there, the nurses . . . The whole *staff*, right through to the helpers. The ladies who run the shop, everybody. They're all helpful.

A central component of the contribution of centre staff apparent in patients' accounts was the cohesiveness of the staff, and the consistency of contact with 'helpful' and knowledgeable people. Patients were often unsure about the reasons for some of the procedures, like the weekly blood sample, and described the technicians as always willing to answer questions, often in technically explicit language. Radiotherapy staff were frequently asked questions about the effects trajectories of treatments, and about what would happen after the treatment calendar finished. This created some problems for staff, who were not 'authorized' to give out such information ('sensitive' information, like whether function loss would be permanent, and information about how a particular patient's treatment calendar would be handled at follow-up). Patients pointed out the difficulty of knowing who was in charge of such information and puzzled over the evasion of some radio-therapy staff in replying to specific questions, when they were generally so informative.

Treatment staff were seen to be conscientious about making referrals to other staff as well as to the consultant if they suspected there were problems in the treatment calendar that might best be dealt with by other agents. Alice, 50, a business owner with breast cancer, had 'pressed' the senior registrar to refer her to the in-house physiotherapist when her arm was still 'frozen' two months following removal of lymph nodes from under the arm:

AW: It were seizing up you see because it . . . you don't know what you *should* be doing, you're afraid to do things. They, they just understand so completely what they're *deal*ing with, without *push*ing you. I couldn't believe how, what a difference it made in such a short time. And then, and they were very open, very chatty. And the physiotherapist asked me if I'd had someone to see that, for sort of support, d'you know what I mean, I don't know what they call them . . . I *had*n't, but I, always felt that I didn't want to talk to anybody *neg*ative so I never pushed it to get involved with anybody, because I've felt I was coping with it well meself. How*ever*, she asked me if I'd like to see this, lady that was, voluntary, which I *did* and, she just *lis*tened to me. And I think at the *time*, you feel so much better if somebody will *lis*ten to you to pour everything out onto, you, you get rid of, the load. She'd had a mastectomy 25 years ago, so you felt that she knew what you were talking about *any*way. *Those* two things I found very *very* helpful.

Another key aspect of patients' voiced satisfaction with the care they received at the centre from lower status staff had to do with a sense of companionship, 'moral support', and interest offered by radiographers and nurses. Gerald, 67, a retired engineer with lung cancer, had an interesting experience when he apparently coughed up a piece of his inoperable tumour at the beginning of his radiotherapy calendar:

> GW: I'd had two treatments, and I was sitting here, Saturday afternoon, and I got a very severe bout of *cough*ing, and *sudd*enly, I got this piece of stuff up, it was about *that* long, about *that* wide and it, at the *end* of it was like the root of a, you know when a tooth's extracted, all with blood on it. And I put it in a bottle. And uhm, un*fort*unately the machine was *off* on the Monday and Tuesday, so it was *Wed*nesday before I took it in, and the radiographers were . . . *oh* and they said, 'That's *wond*erful, never seen anything like *this*', and they took it away. Then the doctor called me in, a young girl, and she said 'Well there's nothing we can do with this, it's been too long away from the blood supply', she says, 'Just take it away.' She couldn't care *less* about it, she wasn't interested. If it had been Dr D [consultant] might have been a different tale. It was still in the *gin*! And *my* own doctor seemed to think it was part of the tumour.

Gerald had been under the care of a homeopath during treatment, and had experienced remarkably few side effects from radiotherapy, despite the sensitive location of the tumour, near his oesophagus. The radiographers had expressed interest in this, and, along with his GP, in his 'Tommy the tumour' (as he called it) experience described above. Feelings of acknowledgement were often described in patients' accounts as a core aspect of the care they were shown by centre staff.

The continuity and supportive contact described above was notably absent from some in-patients' experiences with temporary ward night staff. One of these patients, May, 53, a pub caterer with floor-of-mouth cancer, described a disturbing encounter with one such nurse:

> MS: Well there were an old lady opposite wasn't there? She were a nice old lady but she were *wand*ering a bit. *Oh* and this night, she tried to get out of bed and *I* s'pose she was a bit senile, so I pushed for nurse, and she started *shout*ing at this lady . . . I says, '*Don't* shout at her like that.' '*Ex*cuse me May,' she says, 'are *you* telling me my job?' I says, 'I'm *not*' . . . but it wasn't just her. As one patient at back of me put it, Marion, that girl that was, well she was dying and she was only a young girl, she says, 'They

just don't know what we've to *go* through on a night, they're just
here for a few hours at night and they *see* us curled up in bed
asleep and that's all they're bothered about, that's all they *want*,
a*sleep*, they're all sat in rest room smoking.' 'Cause I used to
have to go to the toilet a lot, they used to let me take me Ensure
[gastric feeding] off and go on me own you know. But we'd to
walk past the rest room and there they were smoking with their
feet up. They want reporting at [the centre] night staff, some of
them.

As described by May, these nurses lacked a real 'stake' in the centre and
work with its patients. She ascribed this to their temporariness (two or
three nights a week were 'covered' by agency nurses). This casual status
seemed to be at the root of the poor care described by several patients who
were in-patients like May for an extended period during treatment.

The lack of a formal, routine 'pick-up' of patients who needed or wanted
special help (like counselling, dietary and wound care advice, physiotherapy)
was discussed by several patients. While identification of special needs was
a part of the routine work of the radiographers and nurses, there was a
good deal of luck involved in patients being identified for help, especially
as patients rarely requested help themselves. The mastectomy counsellor
was a volunteer who had no office from which to work, and who had to
rely on the observations of treatment staff and the waiting areas to identify
patients who needed or wanted her help. The dietitian was a recent addition to the staff at the time of the interviews, and she too had no 'fixed
address' at the centre. There was no routine referral of post-operative
patients to the two resident physiotherapists. Auxiliary staff like these
were thus few and very much peripheral presences at the centre, which
made it difficult for patients to know who to ask for when requesting
'special' help. Below, Abby, 46, a retired NHS manager and nurse with a
new career as a gestalt therapist, commented on what she saw as a gap in
the service at the centre:

> AW: I talked to one woman in particular. We'd followed each other
> through getting set-up and starting treatment, and she was young
> and she, had been diagnosed privately and we were talking about
> counselling, and she'd had no information at all and was *really*
> floundering . . . nobody was picking her up. She was *worried* out
> of her mind. She'd had slight weight loss – well she was post-op
> of course, and they'd asked to do a bone scan – *she* was *past*
> herself. Well she knew one of the complications was bone cancer,
> she'd lost weight so therefore . . . you know, and so, I said, 'Yeah
> I had a bone scan after my mastectomy.' She said, 'Did you?' I
> said, 'Yeah, sometimes they do it sometimes they don't, depends
> on the doctor.' But I thought how sad that nobody's picked her

up. And I suppose to a certain extent, nobody either at [City B hospital] or at [City A centre] is picked up in that way. So . . . nobody's picked up routinely, like, *do* you want to talk, *do* you know what's going on?, and *re*ally sitting you down and telling you what's going on. That actually doesn't happen, there *isn*'t the time. So, yeah, the questions, the information you've pretty much got to have it all in your head.

An implicit treatment calendar task for treatment staff is that of making sure that patients' needs are met with adequate resources, and this involves two complementary tasks: ensuring that resources are not used 'unnecessarily' (and deciding what constitutes justifiable use), and ensuring that those who need certain resources (medicines, time, treatment procedures, transportation, in-patient stay) get them. Nursing and radiography staff showed keen awareness of the tendency for patients *not* to state their needs unequivocally because of a wish not to seem 'ungrateful' or complaining, or because of 'not really being ill enough' to warrant attention (prescription nurses commented often about patients who told them about problems they would then deny having in the presence of senior professionals). Ellie, 64, a retired catering assistant, describes being given permission to use resources during her in-patient stay at the centre on an isolation ward for implanted wire treatment:

ER: So one night I lay awake for an hour, and then I put the light on and read for an hour, then put the light off and went back to sleep. So the next morning the nurse came in and said, 'Did you have a good night?' And I said, 'Not *re*ally', and told her, and she said, 'Why didn't you ring the bell?' I only rang it once the whole time I was there. She says, '*Why* didn't you ring the bell? I could have brought you in a cup of tea.' I said, 'Oh, I don't like to bother you because,' I said, 'there's people in here that are *ill*.' You know I think that, 'cause I never think that I were, I wasn't *re*ally ill.

This sanctioning and anticipating of needs is central to the work of treatment and support staff. The 'flip-side' of this work is that of protecting resources that are already stretched. Nurses at the weekly review clinic for example had to ensure the steady flow of patients through the consultant's examining rooms by making sure patients did not stay too long after the 'business' of the examination was over. This meant hurrying some patients along and juggling review times with treatment and other appointments (blood taking or scans for example). The contradictory positions of being an advocate for patients' needs and a provider of resources to satisfy these needs on the one hand, and a safeguarder and restricter of service resources on the other, must be managed by treatment staff on a daily basis. Within the context of the clinic, the needs of patients and those of the service itself are not always consonant. The work of treatment staff in managing this situation as part of treatment schedule management gives a view of the treatment calendar as an arena in which resources are competed for by patients and professionals, and in which 'moral adequacy' (Silverman 1985) must at all times be addressed and defended by patients, and acknowledged in the work of staff.

Senior treatment calendar professionals and treatment calendar management

Once a treatment calendar is set up, the management work of senior professionals is generally simplified, until follow-up to the treatment calendar begins (which may of course bring more and/or different treatments to the treatment calendar). Calendar management becomes more complex for patients who become terminally ill and require palliative *care* as well as treatment, and for those who are being treated with more than one mode within several treatment calendars. Also, those who are dealing with another major illness or condition besides the cancer will have complicated illness calendars, as will those who are being treated in more than one institution. Sometimes all the above conditions may apply to a single individual.

During the initial radiotherapy and chemotherapy calendars, the business of treatment calendar management is similar for senior professionals as for lower status professionals: monitoring patients' reactions to treatment (in terms of side effects) and ensuring that they complete the treatment calendar as planned, if at all possible. In addition, they must decide whether the original treatment trajectory has changed, and alter the treatment calendar accordingly (like adding chemotherapy sessions to an existing schedule, or deciding against implanted wire treatment in favour of chemotherapy if metastases are discovered). Treatment calendar management during a first schedule of treatment consists of arranging for the management of side effects and seeing that the treatment calendar is completed as planned, or altered as appropriate.

The weekly treatment review was the usual context of interaction of senior professionals with patients. Most patients described the reviews as perfunctory, or as just another routine in the treatment calendar (that could add one to two hours to a treatment day). It seemed in part the sense of knowing the treatment calendar manager as a *person* that made the review significant for some patients. In these instances, being treated as an 'individual' (a pervasive conceptualization in the biomedical model of the patient as a 'case' distinct from other 'cases') had seemed to become being treated as a 'person'.

Still, the majority of patients described feeling rushed through the treatment review, finding it difficult to recall questions, as Kevin, 60, an unemployed security officer with floor-of-mouth cancer and leukaemia, recalls:

KC: It never seemed appropriate to ask the doctors questions at the time when they were *there*. You know it, things that you wanted to know, things that came to mind, while they... they weren't *there* as soon as they were there, my mind went blank.

Of particular difficulty was the shortness of time available for the review (around five minutes per patient), and the fact that one of several professionals could be in attendance (consistent contact with one central person was not assured), including people the patient had never seen before. A general feeling of having to piece together information from overheard technical discussions was present in patients' accounts of encounters with senior professionals, as Francesca describes:

FA: They don't tell you an *aw*ful lot at hospital. Bits of it, me daughter-in-law could tell me, you know with being a nurse... I know I sort of, you hear them, talking amongst themselves when you first go and they're marking you up and all that. They were deciding how to place me leg because Dr D said, 'We don't want to do, *too* much in your leg because it'll just, just destroys, cells we don't *want* destroying.' So, they were sort of, he was saying, 'We'll do it *this* way and twist the leg so-and-so so it just goes down there you know and...', he sort of basically what you heard them say be*tween* them, that you pick bits up don't you. I mean they don't really sit down and *tell* you, properly. I don't... mind you then again, they've probably haven't the time to go into details I don't know. They always seem so rushed don't they? You know, I don't know.

In addition to a lack of direct discussion with professionals and the shortness of consultations, contact with professionals who did not know one could create problems. Such encounters left the patient vulnerable to suddenly being seen (defined) differently from the way they had been with their 'regular' radiotherapy consultant or senior registrar, as Abby, 46, a former nurse and NHS manager with breast cancer, describes:

AW: So when I saw the doctor, he said, 'How are you?' I said, 'Well, actually I'm *fine*, but last night I hit the wall of tiredness for the first time, but that's OK'. And I promptly got a lecture on thinking *positively*. I said, '*That's* got nothing to do with it,' I said, 'you asked me how I felt, and I have felt tired, and that's OK'. He said, 'Well you've got to think more positively, about your dis*ease*!' And I thought, *next* time, if I see you again sunshine you'll get nothing from me. But I didn't see him again, and actually last week Dr D asked me, 'How are you feeling', and I said, 'Fine, but I've had the occasional wall of tiredness', and he said, 'Yeah, you're bound to', and that was *fine*! That was all I'd wanted.

Patients like these did not see a regular treatment manager each week; their management was handled between the consultant and senior registrar, or between two cities, or both (and there was a certain amount of 'back and forth' management in many treatment calendars). For them, ideas about follow-up, the future treatment calendar, prognosis, and the trajectory reasoning of professionals were much more vague. Here Betty, 44, a retired WREN with breast cancer, voices the concerns of many patients about the significance of the weekly and monthly reviews, and the shape of the unknown follow-up calendar to come:

> *BG:* You don't like to say, 'Well then,' you know, 'is it all *gone*?' I mean I, one doesn't know the *system*, you know and, but I think next time I go for chemotherapy, I'll say, 'At what *stage* are you able to say, it's all gone, or it's still *there*, or, you know, what's going on *inside*?' I mean I haven't got a *clue* what's going on. 'Cause I know that when all the treatment's finished you have to be assessed you know every three months six months and once a year and, all that, but how do they *know*? I mean, oh it's all right when you're having the radiation 'cause you've got the whole *pic*tures, the images. They can see but, when you're having chemotherapy you're having a drug, shot into your . . . my *fix* as they call it, every three weeks. How do they know what's going on? I mean I know that chemotherapy is only a pre*cau*tion. I mean it might be . . . I mean *I* don't want all the, the *gory* medical details but I mean, you know. I just want to know if I'm, for me own peace of *mind* I mean, I don't know anymore I haven't a clue what's going on in there.

Patients did not receive the information they said they most wanted at reviews, namely, whether they still 'had cancer', and how serious their prognostic situation was, largely because not much was known by professionals at this time, the results of treatment and surveillance scans taking time to assess. This was a frustrating situation, and one they described not feeling able to confront in the weekly review with the senior professional. But in addition to the (often overwhelming) issue of disease status, basic problems of function, side effects, and how to live life in treatment went unacknowledged in many a review encounter. Here Rachael, 41, a supply teacher with breast cancer, describes the limbo of the treatment situation:

> *RS:* *No* I mean most people say to me, 'Well how are you? Are you *bett*er now, have you got the all-clear?', but, I don't suppose you

ever *do* do you? You know maybe that . . . you just keep going back and having check-ups. I'm not, didn't get it *per*sonally but they probably wouldn't *give* me any tests unless, you have a mammograph.

A central problem here was that patients had received no information about how follow-up would be managed and disease status assessed. At times, the treatment review process could seem quite chaotic. Alice, 50, a business owner with breast cancer, describes the inconsistency arising from the difficulties of being given chemotherapy treatment at the referring hospital in City B by the centre's radiotherapy consultant's senior registrar, while seeing the consultant at the centre for radiotherapy reviews and sometimes for chemotherapy treatments and reviews at both the centre and the City B hospital:

> AW: I'll tell you something else as well. The first day that I saw *you* at [the centre] which is eight weeks ago, my *hus*band was there, and Dr D told me that it was in *all* the glands and that I would have to have eight lots of chemotherapy, and seven weeks after that, he asked me if there was anything I was *wor*ried about and I said the only thing that I would *worry* about was that, I can't accept that it was in all the glands and it hasn't gone *fur*ther, and he said it *was*n't in all the glands, only two. And I think the worst *time* for me was coming away after he told me that it was in all the glands, and for him to *say* that it *was*n't, after seven weeks I thought that was a bit rich. *Al*so I went to [referring hospital in City B] *six* weeks later for, supposedly chemotherapy treatment, I'd just had an appointment card to see *him*, and he'd said, 'We'll see Dr L [surgeon] and Dr LA [radiotherapy senior registrar] will be with me and we'll all have a *chat*.' When I arrived there was only *him* there and he said something about, 'Your blood count's down you can't have the chemo today', I said I didn't know I was *hav*ing chemo today. He said, 'What do you think you're *here* for?' He said, 'It would have been your last.' And I said I understood I have another three *months* to come, he said, 'Oh no, it'll be the *last*.' And so, he'd *told* me two conflicting *dif*ferent *tales*, and I'd had the *worry* of it because I felt it was much worse than it ended up *being*.

Possibly as a result of patchy information management, information from the consultant at different stages of the treatment calendar was contradictory and the follow-up procedure after radiotherapy quite different from what had been discussed earlier. The chemotherapy treatment calendar (and prognostic implications) was also given a different reading by the consultant at follow-up than that heard by Alice and her husband at the outset of the radiotherapy and chemotherapy treatment calendars. Abby also experienced repeated difficulties with key professionals' management of her 'case':

AW: That's it, being believed. Dr D hadn't written down on my sheet had he? So I went to the radiographer and he wrote down 15, I said, 'No, no it's 20.' He said, 'Well he hasn't written it down and it's usually 15.' So the next time I went to review clinic and asked Dr D, and he said, 'No, technically it's 15 and 5, so 20 altogether. 5 booster.' And he *still* didn't write it on my notes. The week be*fore* I saw Dr F [registrar] and he said, 'Well you're finished.' I said, 'No, I've got another 5', 'No,' he said, so he then made a telephone call – and all because it hadn't been written in my notes! Now again, if this hadn't been *me*, who *knows* what would have happened? This has been the whole pattern for me – me filling in gaps.

Abby described the frequent oversights she experienced as a result of shared management of her case by several professionals, and a failure of several to keep up with the 'details':

AW: They actually don't read the notes. They actually do not read what's written. 'Cause when I had this second lump this time, it was really debatable whether I *would* have radiotherapy. [They said] 'We don't *usu*ally do this on a new metastatic wound site', I said, 'Yes, but that site is three and a half years old'. [They said], 'Yes but it says on the *wound* site', I said, 'Well I've had another lump removed' . . . They don't read what's *there*.

A serious problem for many patients was the surgical follow-up appointment (usually three months post-operatively), at which they had expected to see the surgeon, senior registrars and/or diagnosing consultant, but were faced instead with an unknown 'doctor'. Francesca, 67, a housewife with a thigh sarcoma, describes the futility of such a visit:

FA: Well I went last Tuesday, to [City A hospital], as *I* thought to see Mr L [surgeon], but it was another chap I've never ever *seen* before now that when I was *in* hospital but, and he didn't say his *name* they usually say, 'Oh I'm, doctor so-and-so', and he, examined it but it was swollen with treatment and he said, 'Well I can't really tell, tell you anything', he said, 'you better come back in another three weeks.' And see I'm *hop*ing I see Mr L next time he said Mr L was away . . . I'd never ever seen him, don't know haven't a *clue* who he was. Didn't hear anyone say his *name*, he seemed to be in such a hurry and there were that many and they kept bringing him out of clinic to go down to another room and then he'd come back and then they'd fetch him again I thought oh *God* we're never going to get *seen* to you know. He just sort

of had a look, he said, '*Oh* well it's still swollen I can't really tell.'
I'd *nev*er ever seen him. I thought he, I know he's all me notes
and I've a *stack* of notes. He was sort of flicking through 'em but
they can't digest it all in a few minutes can they really, what all's
been done, what things there are?

The busyness of the clinic, the frequent interruptions, the fact that neither
Francesca or the registrar know who they are talking to all undermine the
purpose of the review. The result is wasted time for both the clinic and
Francesca. In addition, her rehabilitation needs go unaddressed (her swollen
leg is itself a significant problem for her) and she gets no advice or help in
dealing with these function problems arising from surgery and exacerbated
by radiotherapy. Rachael describes a similar experience:

RS: When I went to see Mr H [surgeon], oh I can't remember how
      long ago it was, I'd just been out of hospital [the centre, follow-
      ing implanted wire treatment] maybe a couple of weeks. But you
      see he just seemed very busy and tired, and kept putting his hand
      on the doorknob and I kept asking another question! And then
      he'd turn round and answer me but, I felt as if I didn't have,
      enough time, to talk about little things, which probably were not
      important, but I came out feeling quite angry with him . . . just how
      long it would take for my, breast to seem . . . it still seems *swoll*en,
      how long would it take that, to disappear. Swimming, things like
      swimming you know, things you can use on your skin, *di*et, you
      know should you have, still continue with more of a high-protein
      diet, to boost your blood cells or, you know *li*ttle things.

Chaotic follow-up (a lack of consistency of contact, and of information)
was an all-too-familiar experience described in patients' accounts. Phil,
58, a bait farm worker with terminal lung cancer, and his wife had been
concerned about if and when a new radiotherapy calendar would begin, as
Christmas was approaching, and preparations would have to be made if
Phil had severe side effects to deal with over the holidays:

PH: I passed him [radiotherapy consultant] in the corridor [of the
      City A referring hospital], so they must, you know must go
      down to the [referring hospital] later in the day, 'cause he has a
      clinic there every Tuesday, and, even though I didn't *see* him,
      because uh, what happened there had been an emergency, and
      he'd been called out and of course this young, young one said
      you know Dr S [senior registrar] is busy, and Dr D [consultant]
      is being called out on an emergency. So he went to confer with
      Dr S when he'd examined me chest and that and then come back
      and told me that they'd be sending a card to go up to [City A
      centre] for some further treatment you know.

Phil describes being left with no real answer to his question of when the further treatment will begin, so that he and his wife can plan their personal calendar accordingly. In contrast, those few accounts that detailed instances of direct and decisive communication, though often about difficult realities like permanent loss of function from treatment, were described as 'satisfying', in that patients had an issue of importance to them acknowledged. Here May, 53, a pub caterer with floor-of-mouth cancer, describes a post-radiotherapy review at the centre:

> MG: Dr D told me, 'We've no . . .', he didn't even *think* about it, he just says, 'and you'll get your taste back in about three months *fully*', 'cause that's what I were frightened of. They've all been a bit, when I've asked them at [the centre], Sister she, they were all a bit *strange* they didn't want to *an*swer me, and I thought, are they telling me I'm going to be like *this* rest of me *life* you know. Well it really upset me did that. No taste – it's a terrible thing, and then when I had, well I didn't *have* to ask Dr D, it upset . . . *well* he *did*n't upset me he just said, 'At first you shall *nev*er be able to eat anything dry on, the tongue and you'll *al*ways have to have a drink with you wherever you go,' he said, 'because I *don*'t think we can get your saliva back.' Took it here with me tongue and me throat you see. He said, 'You *might* just get it back a bit on *this* side but I don't know.' He says, '*But*, your *taste*,' – I didn't even ask him about me taste but he says, 'you'll get it back in three months *fully*.'

Here both good and bad news forms a mixed offering (and directness is always easier when there is good news to impart), but May describes coming away with a clear picture of her functional situation that puts at least some of her concerns to rest.

As well as the lack of consistency of contact with central treatment professionals that could so often plague reviews, patients' lack of knowledge about how disease status was assessed (and when), and the significance of test results, were frequently neglected concerns. Larry, 70, a retired factory foreman with terminal lung cancer, describes apparently getting lost in the shuffle upon completion of his palliative radiotherapy course:

> LH: Me doctor [senior registrar] said, as far as she was concerned, I'd had me treatment, and she's passing me back to him [diagnosing consultant], and he [radiotherapy consultant] said, 'Have you got an appointment?' I said, 'No', he said, 'We'll make one for you.' I've heard nothing since that was, what six or seven weeks ago?
>
> Wife: He's supposed to give him some x-rays to see how things has worked.

LH: That's what I *think* they are – they haven't, see I haven't had any since I had the treatments. Well I, the day I came out I had some x-rays I had x-rays and then came out, but I think the idea is that you know he's going to see me and they should have some *more*. So I don't know, that's one thing they didn't tell me. I mean Dr D seemed to be, you know rushed off their feet as they are so I, I mean there were huge queues when I went to see her [senior registrar] and uh, I waited about an hour and a half to be told that she was, handing me over to Dr H and that was it, nurse said, 'Don't go undress' [laughs].

Reviews of treatment were often described as superficial, with little explicit technical discussion from professionals. Below, Francesca describes a surgical review after the completion of her radiotherapy calendar:

FA: They must have been scan pictures, and they had all these little pictures clipped up on a board, it were first time I'd seen them. And of course I was sort of . . . not that I knew *really* what they were but I could sort of, had a *vague* idea looking at 'em. And when I got outside again afterwards after he'd seen me, I were telling me daughter-in-law and I said, 'Oh you'd have known Maureen!' She says, 'Oh I wished I'd seen them', she says, 'I nearly come in with you.' You know you don't know whether doctors like, somebody coming in with you . . . She says, 'Oh I nearly asked if I could come in', I says, 'I never thought to,' I said, 'they ought to come out' 'cause they were, they stuck these pictures and lit 'em up like and then of course they all disappeared [surgeon and senior registrar] and I were waiting for the doctor coming, she could have come in and looked while we were waiting for the doctor!

Patients described feeling unwilling or incapable of directly questioning professionals about follow-up and disease status. They described using a mixture of direct questioning and drawing their own conclusions on the basis of professionals' 'manner', and unsolicited remarks. Bronwyn, 58, a housewife with cancer of the chortoid, describes piecing together her own hopeful prognostic view in such a way:

BG: We've been back to see Mr N, like the consultant, and uh he did say that we did the right thing taking your eye out Mrs G 'cause he said three, four more days and they wouldn't have been able to do anything for me so I said *oh* thank you very much, I couldn't thank him *enough*. I did say to that girl [senior registrar] yesterday that doctor, 'Am I clear?' So she said, 'We as*sume* you are but it's . . .'. She said I could come back in three months, and, they'll keep an eye on me . . . But she seemed *happy* about me you know, 'cause you can tell when they talk to you *you* know, she said if I want to discuss . . . when I was having all this pain she was, seemed a bit, concerned you know. And that's when she sent me for this scan and, he even scanned me *eye* [removed eye] on its *own*, sent it, in this thing, you know, but they said it was all for, teaching you know.

Treatment and post-treatment reviews can be threatening situations, and many patients described fearing that they would hear 'bad news' if they asked too many questions.

As time went on, however, the issues of disease status and prognosis could become more pressing, particularly as most patients were aware that the surveillance schedules they were often subjected to were there to provide information about these crucial issues, although this information was frequently not shared explicitly with the patient. Surveillance was often handled by professionals the patient had never met before, a factor that could complicate the communication of serious information, about the presence of metastases for example, as Melissa, 49, a university housekeeper with breast cancer, describes:

MG: Well he just sort of said, he tested me and what-have-you and said that they'd found a couple of spots at the top on my *spine*, I said, 'Well I understand that that could be something to do with ar*thri*tis that I had.' So he said, 'Oh,' he said, 'it might *not* be, you know I don't *know*.' So I just said, 'Oh', you know I just left it at *that*, and then when we went in to see Dr L [senior registrar] she explained that she didn't think it *was* the arthritis she thought it was, you know a couple of spots from the *can*cer, which as *she* said, we *can't* cure it, but it can, be treated with radiotherapy.

Husband: But I think that Dr L was surprised we didn't know this, from the previous . . . talking to the previous doctor. She says, 'You don't *know*?' So we just said, 'No.'

It is precisely at such 'sensitive' points in the treatment calendar (when prognosis is reassessed) when consistent contact with one or two central treatment professionals is most important. A dependable relationship with key professionals lays the groundwork for difficult subsequent encounters, when 'bad news' may have to be discussed.

Managing effects – the treatment work of patients and close others

Strauss and colleagues since 1975 (Strauss and Glaser 1975; Strauss *et al.* 1985; Corbin and Strauss 1988) have applied ideas from the sociology of work to the experience of illness. These authors investigated the management of chronic illness in acute care institutions (Strauss and Glaser 1975), pointing out that much illness management work performed in the hospital is managed by patients and their families (Strauss *et al.* 1985), and chose to explore the management of chronic illness by patients and spouses at home (Corbin and Strauss 1988). This work highlights the issue of resources (time, energy, money) in the management of illness and treatment. Part of the work of patienthood is that of 'calculating resources', and 'maintaining a relative balance in the distribution and utilisation of resources among illness, biography, and everyday life work involves continual calculation of resources' (Corbin and Strauss 1988: 118). The excerpts from patients and spouses that follow here reflect how treatment and personal calendar management is bound up with the management of resources, both for the individual patient and family, and the community, including health professionals and treatment institutions.

The experienced effects of radiotherapy and chemotherapy (in addition to those from unresolved post-surgical problems) and the impact of the treatment calendar itself bring about the erosion of the lifespace of the ill person, through the draining away of time and energy from the personal calendar.[1] This impact is made worse by the effects of disease itself (although for many patients initially, this is the least difficult aspect of the illness calendar experience). The struggle to meet the aims and goals of the illness calendar (which displace those of the personal calendar) causes an erosion of the lifespace. This displacement of the personal and life calendars is arguably the single most important 'effect' (in terms of quality of life) on the ill person of treatment, the treatment calendar, and the disease process.

The extent (and duration) of this taking-over of life by illness and medical agendas depends on a range of factors, including the stage of illness, type of treatment calendar(s) involved, and the life circumstances (from age to socio-economic status) of the ill person. Gary, 60, a plumber with terminal mesothelioma (asbestos cancer), describes the 'loss of grip', both physical and mental, that advanced illness and the effects of prolonged treatments (some of which are to control the effects of *other* treatments) have wrought in him:

> GL: Another thing hurts me and that's, it's progressing *worse*r. There's less I can *do*, forge*t*ful, can't think from one minute to next, memory's *gone* and I can't *hold* owt, *drop* all sorts, every cigarette, couple of seconds on the floor. I'll be sat like that in chair and it's *gone*, just like that, no *grip*, just can't hold *on* to anything.

In being both unable to remember things, and unable physically to grasp objects, Gary describes how, through the disease and treatment, he is losing his 'grip' on his daily existence, on his life in general. On a general level, such losses affect the individual's ability to 'pass the time' meaningfully, as

Terry, 64, a retired electronics technician with larynx cancer, and his wife describe:

Wife: You can't *leave* him any more he's not much patience.
TL: No, I haven't been able to *con*centrate much.
Wife: And he was, buying books with crosswords in you know. Doesn't have patience to do all that.
TL: It hasn't been a brilliant week. I've done a little pottering around in the garden a bit but uh, in fact I think apart from reading newspapers I can't read that much and I've been too *tired* to be bothered with anything like that. Waiting for tomorrow, I shall feel better when I've got this [post-radiotherapy review] over.

Treatments and medications frequently have an undermining effect on the capacity to *live* in the personal calendar (to act, think and experience), and this compromised ability to engage with the personal calendar begins to characterize experience within the treatment calendar as treatment (and sometimes the disease itself) progresses. Adam, 58, a retired textiles worker with lung cancer, describes the suspended animation of each day spent dealing with the enervating impact of radiotherapy:

AL: I was uh, I was all right for a couple of hours after the treatment and, after that I were just drained. It knocked the life . . . I had to lay down I couldn't sleep. I slept all right when I went to *bed*, but during the afternoon and evening, while the effects were there I couldn't keep me eyes open but, still I couldn't sleep I was just drained. I was just shattered from head to foot, which you know, they said, it affects different people different ways. I mean I used to talk to a chap that were only having two fields when I were having three but . . . it had taken him off his food, he wasn't eating, he felt sickly with it and that sort of thing but I've never felt sickly with it, which was a big advantage. I found it *hard*, not saying I didn't. I mean at that stage, for them few hours, a bit depressing. I don't get depressed, but I think it were a depression that was *brought* with the treatment you know it wasn't there before or since.

A major impact of treatment substances (for example, radiation or drugs) is that of undermining the identity of the ill person, making him or her less *like* (recognizable as) him or herself. Adam describes radiotherapy as 'knocking the life' out of him; May, 53, a pub caterer with floor-of-mouth cancer, said that morphine made her 'like a dead person', so that she could not communicate with her family at visiting hours; Minnie, 80, a housewife with cancer of the anal margin, found that antibiotics for an infection left her confused and inarticulate, 'as if I was drunk' (possibly an allergic reaction, or an interaction between the antibiotics and other medications and chemotherapy drugs). One of the paradoxes of medicine is that the procedures and substances used to treat disease often produce problems (requiring treatment) all their own.

The 'side' effects of treatments may be such that patients opt to cut them out altogether, preferring to deal with pain rather than continue to suffer the unwanted effect. Here Bertha, 62, with metastatic breast cancer, describes taking such measures:

> BB: I'm not happy about the morphine – I try to avoid it at all costs! The morphine makes me nauseous, so they give me matirium to stop that. And when I take the matirium I get indigestion! So, I was getting this terrible indigestion, and it stopped when I stopped taking the matirium and morphine!

Kevin, 60, a former security officer with floor-of-mouth cancer and leukaemia, also describes finally taking matters into his own hands, at a suggestion from a treatment centre nurse:

> KC: Well the *worst* side effect, and it's only just cleared up last week, was uh, consti*pa*tion. And I went four weeks without going to the *toi*let, and when I *told* 'em about it last week when I went to see the specialist I expected 'em *do*ing something or saying something like, but I never got in and out with anything. I'm on, morphine and sulphate, I *was* taking it four times a day. Happens that the lady there [nurse] just said cut it *down*, but they didn't say I'd got to by how *much*. And I just sorted me own mind well, I'll cut it down to nothing if, *ne*cessary, cause I felt *so* dreadful I was upsetting people left right and centre.

Dealing with more than one major treatment calendar (radiotherapy and chemotherapy) run concurrently brings the added difficulty of compounded effects of the different treatments. Betty, 44, a retired WREN with breast cancer, describes the uncertainty of predicting how each phase of treatment will affect her, as the effects from one treatment complicate those from another:

> BG: I mean one doesn't know what to ex*pect* as I said to my, GP yesterday. But, all I wanted to do when I'd been given it [chemotherapy] is to get *home* and, you know *sit* and relax. And *basic*ally you're sat there thinking now, what's going to happen *this* time? Because now I've had *three* I compare the symptoms, and how I felt after each one. But there a*gain* you see this one was the *first* one after all the radiation had been finished. Because I was, feeling very sick and that, from the radi*a*tion, and my stomach and everything had settled *down*, and I'd had about

> ten days after radiation had finished before I had the chemo on *Thurs*day so it was going to be interesting from that point of *view*, which was sparking, reacting on the other.

The effects of treatments are often hard to separate and most treatment calendars involve dealing with the effects of a treatment which is itself addressing the effects of another treatment, and so forth.

The impact of 'side' effects of treatment on identity was heard to be quite dramatic, not just in terms of how effects impacted on functioning, but also in terms of the redefinitions of personal identity they seemed to represent for many patients. May describes her shock at reading the report attached to her bed when she was admitted as an in-patient towards the end of her radiotherapy treatment calendar:

> *MS:* They put me on the ward straight off, to day and *night* on that 'Ensure' [gastric feeding] you know. But I was crying when I looked at report, she had me down for, must be fed – malnu*tri*tion and dehydration, I could've dropped through the floor, I mean you don't think in this day and age do you, malnutrition?

This redefinition brought about by the realization that frightening and alien-sounding diagnostic labels suddenly apply to oneself is reflected in the filling-out of forms required to receive benefit. This is often an onerous task for patient and family, particularly as the disease progresses. One form, for money from a DSS 'Special Fund' for terminally ill patients is headed: 'Must have six months or less to live.' Aside from the fact that it is not possible to predict with certainty how much time a patient 'has left', the ill person must face seeing such a label when they fill in the form, and in effect commit themselves to being so bracketed. Abby, 46, a former nurse and NHS manager with metastatic disease (a diagnosis not revealed to her until after interviewing for our study was completed; she had been told she had a local recurrence of breast cancer, though evidence of metastatic spread was noted in her records from the time of her initial diagnosis in 1987), found the label 'carcinomatosis' in her notes literally 'sickening'. She had known patients with this diagnosis and did not look or feel as they had done. She was leading a busy social and work life as a writer and therapist and found the constant renewal of sick notes a reminder of this label and its implications.

The daily work of the treatment centre outpatient clinics in treating the effects of treatment added significantly to the amount of time patients and family members spent in the daily treatment calendar. Terry, 64, a retired electronics technician with larynx cancer, and his wife describe the pervasiveness of effects management:

> *TL:* Well the snag was at the back end of treatment 'cause I was having the booster treatment, I were getting *two* treatments on

two machines. So I was *wai*ting for one machine and then waiting for the other one, each time I went you know.

Wife: You could see the doctor in between right way round, but the minute you get in, well you'd to see the nurse, to get it dressed because it was so bad. Then we'd to wait to see the nurse didn't we? Then when he came out from seeing the nurse, all wrapped up tight . . .

TL: What a mess . . . My *shirt* was rubbing on it, pyjamas was rubbing them . . .

Wife: Sheets, it were on the sheets and the pillowcases because it was, well it's with all the cream wasn't it as you went along. *Plast*er it on, three times a day.

Extensive radiotherapy can lead to other treatment calendars in the form of in-patient stays, physiotherapy, skin care regimens, regimens for pain control and other side effects. These in turn can have *their* effects, such as bile production from prolonged gastric feeding resulting in putrid discharges, and breathing problems, nausea and chronic constipation from morphine. Patients often have to search out solutions for effects' problems, gauging which is the best advice to follow. Here Liam, 73, a retired dental technician with a recurrence of throat cancer, describes finding the best solution to his swallowing problem:

LC: At the hospital, I couldn't swallow. I mentioned it to the doctor, and he said, 'Take some aspirin, three aspirin before you eat.' Well that's all right, but three aspirin before every meal, that's twelve a day! And, they were making me ill you see. So I went to me own doctor and he said, 'We'll take you off those', and gave me some, what you call it, it's like thick cream, white, and that, fortunately after that I was all *right*!

Seeking help with the emotional impact of treatment was a priority for several women patients, who wanted to spare their family members the strain of coping with *their* emotions over diagnosis and treatment. Here Ellie, 64, a retired catering assistant with breast cancer, describes her attempt at managing in this way:

ER: I've been to see my GP *twice*. I went the first day I came out of hospital, because I was a bit shattered. And I went to have a word with *him* and he gave me some tablets, to calm me down. But anyway, when I was in hospital, I'd taken two, one or two every day the whole time, and then when I went in hospital I took them with me 'cause they always want to know what kind of tablets you're taking. I was already taking the Tamoxifen every day. I *show*ed them and she said, '*oh*,' she said, 'I wouldn't bother to take them any more.' She said, 'All they do is slow

your pulse down' . . . I think it was psychological, the thought
that . . . if he's given me a box of *Smart*ies, it was just the fact
that you think something's making you feel better. I was very
mixed up with my feelings and I didn't want to, I didn't *want* to
be upset, because I didn't want to upset the *fam*ily.

Francesca, 67, a widowed housewife with a thigh sarcoma, describes
how effects management could be complicated by centre shutdowns and
lack of transport:

FA: Then when I finished treatment the nurse said, '*Oh* now you're
finished put zinc castor oil on', so she gave me some tubes of
that. Now *I* felt, that that made them scab over more, as though
it was drawing them all the time and just seemed to *keep* scab-
bing and coming off and, so I stopped *us*ing it. Trouble is, I've
run out of me hydro-cortisone, and I, you know I thought oh
gosh *Mon*day, they're not *there*, Tuesday, I rang up yesterday
morning somebody said they were *work*ing yesterday so I rang
up but of course they weren't *work*ing, so I had some Savlon I've
been using, last night and this morning. I will have to ring up and
see if they'll give me it, I don't know. It's just going up on bus,
sitting on bus! [laughs] It's not very comfy! I mean you can't
really sit with your legs stuck out on bus! I'll have to ask them
will you drop me a tube off!

The treatment calendar was extended into what was left of personal calendar
time through the impact of treatment's effects and the time spent trying to
manage them.

Self-management usually involved the help of family members, whose
lives were also dominated by the ill person's treatment effects. Here Gary
describes how he and his wife try to work out the amount and timing of
his medication to control his pain:

GL: The pain is still there, it's stopping me from, I aren't controlled.
I've tried different combinations for it. Alma me wife and me*self*
we've, we've come to this balance of so many, *mor*phine pills,
that's all. Me antibiotics, I'm on a course of antibiotics *they* seem
to do me some good, I got those through the GP . . . the *maj*or
thing is, getting to *sleep*. They haven't come up with anything
on the sixty-thousand dollar question when I can *sleep* the whole
night. You know I'm slowly winning because I found out the combination of these here drugs, is letting me have the odd hour, *so*
hopefully I . . . pulling it out will make me sleep all night *through*.

Terry's wife describes a dramatic experience when Terry began to cough
up a large amount of blood one night in the midst of the radiotherapy
treatment calendar:

Wife: In fact, the first time he was *rea*lly ill and he, got this terrific cough, I went into the bathroom and there was blood *every*-where. It [the centre] was *closed* on the Monday, it was May Day, so we couldn't go until Tuesday, but it was really upsetting was that. It happened three times, but it wasn't as bad the second or third time. I think the first time we were shocked that, we didn't expect it, and the doctor up there, we saw the doctor on Tuesday, he just, said he should have been in hospital *but*, as the *nurse* said, if it's only a small amount of blood it doesn't matter, you can expect it. They explained it *af*terwards. We didn't expect anything like that. I come downstairs after clearing him up and I honestly reckon she didn't *know*, me daughter, from the sight of *me*, 'cause it were a *terri*ble sight.

Gauging the severity of effects and how to deal with them (whether they constitute an 'emergency' and need professional attention) is often a task of spouses or family members. At such times, professional back-up (whether in the form of a district nurse, telephone helpline, or centre nursing staff) is a highly valued support for family members.

There were many examples of the extent of the work performed by patients' family members, both treatment work and that of managing the treatment calendar (working out medication regimens, monitoring the seriousness of effects, arranging for hospital beds, etc.). Relatives' treatment and treatment calendar work was intensive and varied, ranging from dressing burns and preparing special meals, to accompanying patients to treatment and keeping track of treatment calendar details, such as appointment times, and what had been said in each consultation. In addition, they were managing the home (and their own jobs if still employed) and family, often in a context of great disruption caused by the patient's physical suffering.

Patients' management of all the effects of treatment involves management of their impact on the personal calendar with no real knowledge of when functioning will normalize, and ordinary life resume. Adam describes this situation, definitive answers to which are not forthcoming at the post-radiotherapy review:

AL: Although the treatment did *affect* me throat which they said it *would* do, but that will clear up again. But I just feel as I told Dr L [senior registrar] the other day when I was there I just feel as if when I'm swallowing my pipe is, a lot narrower than what it used to be, which she says basically that that could be correct but it . . . you know it'll, it'll come normal again. The *num*ber of things that is going to come *nor*mal again, it's unbelievable!

Establishing what the precise impact of treatment has been on functioning, and which losses can be recouped when, is a frustrating process, as such assessments can take a long time to establish. Even apparently 'minor' function problems can have a dramatic effect on a person's ability to live daily life, and not knowing the recovery trajectory is often an exasperating condition of life in the cancer illness calendar, as illustrated by Francesca's account of radiation burns:

> *FA:* I did ask one of the radiographers how long, because thinking it were just sort of like badly sunburned, how long *that* would last and they said well, *u*sually takes about a fortnight to go away. And then a week last Friday I were talking to one of the nurses while I were getting dressed I said, '*Oh* it is *sore* me leg', and I thought she were joking at first she said, 'Oh it will get worse before it gets *bet*ter' . . . But I think probably it's made it worse because well, when you sit or when you lay you're just continually rubbing it all the time, don't matter what I *do* you see . . . on a night when I'm on me own I always go and get undressed, put me dressing gown on and put all me things up and leave it sort of exposed you know let air get to it.

The impact of some 'side' effects can affect the person's ability to enjoy the taken-for-granted pleasures of living, and this impact of treatment is made more difficult by the uncertainty of if and when functional losses will be recouped, and to what extent a 'normal' life will be possible. Here May, 53, a pub caterer with floor-of-mouth cancer, describes her loss of taste to radiotherapy:

> *MS:* It's like chewing paper, it's what it tastes like. Even some *now*, some of it, mashed po*ta*toes I've no taste at all with them. And that fish, it were beautiful I'd done it in milk, but it hadn't a lot of taste. Now to*ma*to *soup*, or tomatoes, only tomatoes there isn't, it's a taste all its own, I can taste *that*, quite well. And *choc*olate, although I can't eat . . . I *have* tried little bits of chocolate but it *clogs*. It's horrible for that. But at *first* it was just like eating *pa*per, *oh* it were terrible.

Bronwyn, 58, a housewife with cancer of the chortoid, describes the slow process of recovery during which permanent losses are separated out from those which are only temporary:

> *BG:* I have eventually got better, you know each day over the six weeks. Now I went back *yes*terday, but I didn't see Dr D [consultant] I saw this young lady again, don't know what they *call* her but very nice she was. She was surprised how much hair I had lost, and *she* said it, *might* grow back, but Dr D did say it *would* grow back, so we'll have to wait and see. My skin got very pink, and on the inside of me eye it was *really brown*, as if someone had *caught* me one, and me nose here it, that did all

dry up, and in*side*, but that's cleared. I hadn't lost me eyebrow and me tearducts, they're all right. But *af*terwards I had *all* this bunged up feeling all in me head and I said to Harry, 'I don't think I'll *ev*er feel right while I can get up in the morning and you know, with it clear.' It's just about all gone now and me nose has started to *run* [laughs]. Isn't it good!

Patients receiving palliative treatment described the experience of feeling *better* as a result of radiotherapy, once they had recovered from the initial impact of side effects. Here Larry, 70, a retired factory foreman with inoperable lung cancer, describes dramatic improvement in function following palliative radiotherapy:

LH: Well I came home, and they were, wasn't too bad for the first week and then I had two rough weeks, then I picked up. I mean, I can go down those stairs, twenty or thirty times a *day* now, and I don't puff and pant. Maybe a bit out of breath occasionally, but before I went in I couldn't get up. I had to walk three, four steps and have to stop, then go three four more and stop, then go in the bedroom and grab the oxygen mask. But now, I've never had to send for the doctor.

The main question voiced by these patients was that of how long-term the effects would be, and what would or *could* be done for them when radiotherapy was no longer an option for treatment. Bertha, 62, a retired clerk with metastatic disease, described the benefit from her palliative radiotherapy as disappointingly short-lived:

BB: The only thing I want to know is something they can't tell me! I know what the *out*come is, but what I want to know is, how long will it be? I realize that they can't tell me. I tried to ask Dr P [GP] this, how long it *might* be, how short or, if he had any idea how long. And he said well he had one lady, she had her breast off ten years ago, and she keeps having treatment for the same, problem. And that is the nearest I can get to, shall we say *any* information really. I do find that encouraging to an extent. But I'll tell you what has set me back though. Feeling so great, just after I *had* the treatment, and the short length of time it's sort of *lasted*. Knowing that they, can only give you so many treatments and then it has to take its course, it makes you *won*der, how long they are going to be able to treat you. You see I had visions of it lasting a few *months*, but it didn't. All Dr D said was that he didn't want to give me more treatment at present.

Here Bertha describes wanting some answers about something she acknowledges her doctors cannot ultimately know – an estimate of how much time she has left before the disease 'takes its course'. What she *could* obtain through discussions with professionals is an assurance that there will be treatment (in the form of pain relief and care) right up to the point of her death, and repeated opportunities to voice and discuss her fears and concerns about her disease and treatment with knowledgeable people she can trust. In the absence of categorical answers (rarely possible in chronic illness), such discussions are a crucial aspect of care for the dying patient.

Treatment calendar pervasiveness

The pervasiveness of treatments' effects on the body are bound up with the pervasiveness of the treatment *calendar*. The two are interactive, and it is a mistake to think of them as separate. Saunders's concept of 'total pain' (1989) – suffering on many levels – resonates with the idea advanced in this book, that illness and treatment calendars create much suffering in themselves in addition to that caused by illness and treatment. This suffering we have conceptualized in terms of the pervasiveness of both the somatic effects of treatment, and the effects of the treatment calendar on the personal calendar of the ill person and close others.

The treatment calendar is at its most pervasive when the person has very advanced or terminal illness. It exists at this time in the shape of multiple medication regimens and an ongoing palliation and perhaps recovery treatment calendar (hospice or hospital stays) which will be subject to much alteration as the disease progresses or recedes (and there may be many such ebbs and flows in the 'dying trajectory'). The main challenge to the dying person is to live life before they die, and this can be manifestly difficult, even apart from the somatic limitations imposed by the disease and treatment. Gary, 60, a plumber with mesothelioma (asbestos cancer, always the result of exposure to asbestos), describes how his 'terminal' illness calendar had supplanted all his personal calendar goals. His illness calendar must be seen to include his struggle to win compensation from his employers. His personal calendar plans included moving to another city so his wife could be nearer her relatives, and eventually retiring with her to Spain – both of which were contingent on his winning his compensation case:

> GL: So much *must* be [keeping him awake] all the time worrying me like that. Will I ever *get* settled with the courts, will I have, and will it, settle down with what I've *got* this cancer and, so I can get on *liv*ing a bit. And am I just going to get weaker and weaker in a couple of weeks *snuff* it, you know, that could easily be. I certainly *hope* not. Keep saying I'll *fight* it but, getting awful weak . . . I'll just wait and then they, as soon as anything in mail comes at *all* in relation from, that is the firm that I worked for if I can find any words at *all* to send to solicitor I *will* do just to

sort of jog *their* memories to keep the ball *going* like. But I, I've also not heard any more *from* these [lawyers] you know, if you ring for information and see what's happening, and I mean there's half of your life on the *phone*, what they can do, or what's *happp*ened since, you know, when they last contacted me.

The goals of the illness calendar (somatic and 'symptom' control, and trying to get a court date for his compensation case before death) had *become* the personal and life calendars for Gary. Much of his time was spent dealing or attempting to deal with pain and breathing difficulty, while his legal struggle meant he was quite literally spending half of his life on the phone.

Even for those patients least affected by 'side' effects without such advanced illness and in reasonable general health, the pervasiveness of the treatment calendar was a main source of strain, as indicated by Helen, 63, a housewife with breast cancer, commenting on the hardest aspects of the treatment calendar for her:

HB: It *fills* your whole *life*, it *dominates* everything. This is why I – I feel a bit in *lim*bo in a way, and why I can't really assess *some* things most effectively, because, you know, I'm still in the middle of the *woods* sort of thing... because of what it *is* really, it *brings* it *home*, what it is, it *drags* the whole thing on. Usually when you have an operation you *have* it and you've to come *home* and you recover and that's *it*, but *this* you're sort of you come *home*, and then I've got to come *here*. I mean I can, see the *reason* for it and all that sort of thing you know but, I'm not sort of wishing I hadn't *come*, but at the same time it does sort of drag it on, you're still a *patient*, and, you know ... The stress of *why* I'm coming here and the general feeling of being in limbo and it is a whole new way of *life* this, yes, this form of, everything always comes *af*terwards. You find 'go' and then you *pa-a*-ark! [laughs]. Never knew much about *that* before.

The fact that the personal calendar is taken over to a large extent by the treatment calendar is vividly described here; not merely the resource of time spent in the daily treatment schedule, but having the treatment calendar as the *focus* of every day's activities serves as a perpetual reminder of the cancer. The sense of being overtaken by the goals and aims of the treatment calendar is a major aspect of its pervasiveness, and is something that is likely to increase as time goes on, rather than decrease, as Terry, 64, a retired electronics technician with larynx cancer describes:

TL: I don't know somehow, I wanted to get started, when I first *saw* the specialist I knew there was something wrong and I wanted to get it sorted *out* and then we found out what it was I wanted to get *treat*ment and then *all* of a sudden you seem as if you've got on a *merry*-go-round that you can't get off. You . . . you've *joined* something and you wish to hell you hadn't *joined* you've . . . but, you get *on* it and that's it. And then it seems to go on, and on and on.

Terry had 'gone private' in order to get referred quickly, and thus had committed himself to the illness calendar in a more deliberate way than had the other patients interviewed. Radiotherapy's 'after-effects' and the work of the treatment *calendar* (and its effect on the personal calendar) were described as the most difficult aspects of treatment experience. These aspects interacted, to create a situation in which patients' energy (the amount of which affects the amount and quality of time that can be spent on the personal calendar) was slowly drained (creating the need to withdraw from the personal calendar to an extent). This problem is described by Bronwyn, 58, a housewife with cancer of the chortoid:

BG: The treatment it*self*, was no problem. You know you didn't know you was having anything done and the girls were, really nice. It was *af*ter the treatment. I was poorly wasn't I Marion? I used to get home from the [centre] and go straight to bed you know. Well once I'd had me *sleep* and then by the time, tea-time come I was feeling better and then I would have me next treatment next day and I was back to square one wasn't I?

Efforts to plan ahead so as to limit the impact of the treatment calendar on the personal calendar were often thwarted by the after-effects of treatment, as Betty, 44, a retired WREN with breast cancer, describes:

BG: Well, that's it it takes over com*ple*tely and, you know that's *right* you can't plan. That's why I wanted the morning appointment, that's what I thought, I could do things in the afternoon . . . used to get home, anything from half past ten to twelve o'clock depending on what the machine was doing and then, you know have a cup of coffee and go for a walk in the afternoon, and I don't feel like doing that I'm afraid . . . Sometimes when I, said oh well, I'll go to the supermarket and then suddenly I didn't feel like going, I get annoyed with meself, well I want to *go*, you know me *brain* says, I want to go but me body says you *don't* want to go [laughs]. Well I guess we have to learn, the brain says, lovely afternoon, let's go for a walk down to the shops, halfway down the road my body says no you're not. Then I think *oh why* can't I?

These accounts recall what Jobling calls the 'Sysyphus syndrome' (1988). The Sysyphean nature of both the radiotherapy and the radiotherapy calendar is such that, like Sysyphus, the radiotherapy patient every day pushes the stone up the hill, and each day it rolls back down again. One's life is dominated by the process of going for and returning from treatment, and the effects of the treatment on one's ability to act in the personal calendar. Much of the time not spent in treatment is spent dealing with its effects. Another pervasive strain indicated by Alice, 50, a business owner with breast cancer, is that of 'coping', not 'giving in' to depression, and 'keeping a face on', or being seen to 'cope' well.

> AW: I think it *was* just the long days that you *felt* as though you *nev*er came round all *day*. You were just so *tire*d, and it builds up after so long you get . . . it only gets *worse*. I don't think there was anything . . . I never felt emotional about it. It *hasn't* got me down for one minute I've just kept on top and that and I couldn't expect any more than that. It's more than, I was told to expect. So, when I finished work, last Friday, after the long weekend, I gave *in* to it, and felt I wanted to be *left* to *not* bother with me face and the *hair*, for a couple of days, which isn't me. And the fact that I *did*n't, bother with me face and me hair and, occasionally saw meself in the *mirr*or and thought how *dread*ful I looked, I couldn't *bear*, to carry on doing *that* for long, because you *then* feel ill . . . I think you've got to *push* yourself. *I* felt I had to push meself anyway. Every *min*ute of the . . . of the time I wouldn't want to say different. You know you . . . you just haven't to give *in* to it.

The illness and treatment calendars seemed to call forth a public display of 'coping well' from many patients. It was heard to be important to patients to be seen to be bearing up well, and even to be an exemplary coper: to be uncomplaining, to be grateful, to *show* gratitude, and to reward the attentions of others with bravery and an 'upbeat' presentation of oneself in daily contacts with community members and close others. The care received by patients in the treatment calendar was something they all expressed gratitude for, and the cancer illness calendar as a condition for future life, in the form of regular checks and monitoring by professionals, had a comforting aspect, as described by Helen:

> HB: The *skill* that we got, the looking after generally and I mean that's a *big* thing, and the fact that I'll, be monitored for the rest of my life, and that is a *positive* thing. You know, and I take three pills every morning, one's for blood pressure (laughs) and one's for the malignancy and one's for the *ul*cer.

Summary

Treatment calendars create a toll on the lifespace through the time they take up, in their often changeable and unpredictable nature, and through mismanagement. Such 'costliness' of treatment for the individual patient, in terms of actual physical effects and the impact of treatment substances and processes on the resource of energy, and in the rigours of the treatment calendar, is the main condition impinging on quality of life for patients in treatment.

The social contexts of patients' and professionals' treatment work with the management of, struggle for, and justification of resources within the treatment calendar again highlight the nature of treatment as a social situation. The social experience of treatment is structured by illness and treatment calendars that pose serious constraints on, and have wide-ranging implications for, the other calendars the person is living, and for those of close others and community members (and this involves resources issues for all involved in treatment calendar management). This experience of illness and treatment is a public, as well as a private experience – one in which the patient is continually observed ('under surveillance', both in medical contexts and in the community) – and which implicitly (if not explicitly) demands justification by patients and professionals alike of resources used. For the patient and family, clinicians' time and expertise, and the goodwill, time and other resources offered by close others and community members must be continually acknowledged, and 'deservingness' established. An aspect of the latter condition is the need patients and family members may feel to display 'coping'; to be seen as people who cope well. However, the contexts and processes of the treatment calendar can be a source of support and of genuine social contact for many patients and their families. Resources shortages in these environments (in terms of too little time; lack of continuity in contacts with professionals or the institution(s); not enough space; inappropriate use of space; poor physical environments and so forth) greatly reduce the potential of the contexts of treatment to improve (positively influence) quality of life in treatment. The pressure exerted by a situation of resources shortage is a constant, taken-for-granted feature of the treatment situation, one which constrains and shapes the work done both by professionals and patients. Within the notion of illness as political process (Gerson 1976) rather than deviance or as located entirely within the ill person, personal struggles can and must be seen as located within, shaped by, and contributing to a socially constructed *public* life.

Note

1 We prefer 'erosion' to 'shrinking' (Charmaz 1983) because the former is more evocative of the wearing-down effect of treatment and of the treatment calendar.

6 Discussion

This book has focused on the day-to-day of life in treatment for cancer, with an emphasis on the detail of the treatment calendars of a particular group of patients, and on treatment as social interaction, instead of the passive reception of the substances and procedures that comprise technical biomedical treatment. In this focus, the social world of treatment is seen as dominated by calendar management – both personal and illness – involving the management and justification by patients, families and medical professionals of time, energy and other resources. Resources issues are seen here to link the personal contexts of individuals' personal calendars and treatment calendars with the world of the clinic, defined as a social world, and with the broader contexts of the health service, governmental policy, and biomedicine. Of particular concern here is the lack of justification for an individualistic 'behaviour' (deviance) perspective of treatment and illness experience, within which much that is central to quality of life is neglected.

In Chapter 1, the point was made that while oncologic quality of life assessment appears to place the patient as well as the disease on the biomedical agenda, in using the 'functional living' perspective to conceptualize quality of life, it effectively neglects the *person*. In the discussion provided by this book, the point has been made that the *patient* is still not fully included on the treatment agenda, through insufficient attention to certain quality of care and resources management issues. Patienthood (as illness calendar and treatment calendar management) is central to 'illness-related' quality of life, and can be both a major barrier to, or facilitator of, quality of life enhancement in the chronically ill. In many cases (especially initially) it seems that patienthood is a bigger barrier to quality of life than the disease itself.

Quality of life assessment in oncology originated in ideas about impairment and disability, and their assessment. Within this focus, 'handicap' or social functioning was treated at a very gross level. Ironically, the impact of treatment processes *themselves* on the handicap problem has been seriously underestimated. While cancer treatment *is* necessarily disruptive, time-consuming, invasive and productive of functioning problems, attempts by treatment professionals to minimize this disruption could speak directly to the improvement of quality of life for cancer patients. For example, respect for patients' time; 'filling in gaps' in information about clinic protocol, how follow-up will be managed and of what it will consist; and addressing post-surgical function problems (connecting, in effect, one part of treatment at the hospital with another at the treatment centre) – none of these changes need cost much, but could make an enormous difference to quality of life at the 'handicap' level.

We are not arguing that *all* problems are remediable, at least within existing resources. It might not be possible to hire the counselling staff, dietitians, physiotherapists and social workers to cover completely the needs of all the patients at a large centre like the one featured here, or for each patient to have consistent contact with *one* treatment manager. However, there are problems with time, information gaps, and lack of consistency and continuity in the treatment calendar. The implications of these for the quality of care of cancer patients must be acknowledged for inclusion on the 'balance sheet' of pros and cons when health service reorganizations are being considered. Mechanic (1995: 1492), in his major review of social science work in the areas of health and medicine, points to a need for health professionals to take greater notice of the realities of patients' daily lives when he states that 'a major challenge in the management of illness is to shape the treatment regimen and its implementation in light of the conditions that prevail in the home and at work'. This comment highlights the management function of senior professionals especially within the treatment calendars of individual patients. As an example of the *importance* of this management role to satisfaction with care, a recent study by Fakhoury *et al.* (1996) found that informal caregivers' satisfaction with services for dying cancer patients was mainly determined by 'service characteristics'. Carers were most satisfied with district nurses, who, in addition to spending more time with patients and carers, also played a significant role in coordinating other services and liaising with other professionals (in other words, treatment calendar management). Caregivers valued the district nurses' work in enabling greater coordination of care and provision of home care. Such studies suggest that quality of care may hinge directly upon whether patients and carers experience quality of treatment calendar management, an aspect of which is dependable contact with the same professionals.

What can be seen as a failure of quality of life work to deal adequately with the contexts and processes of patienthood (and thus with many quality of care issues) has come about partially as a result of a narrow fascination with measurement and reductionist perspectives in quality of life research. An obsessive focus on measurement, paired with a dominant concern with establishing the responsivity of measures (their ability to distinguish one treatment from another, or one group of patients from another) has obscured much *shared* experience that is central to quality of life in treatment. The focus on measurement as the only means to determine valid knowledge is a result of a spurious scientism evidenced in quality of life and psychosocial oncology, fed in recent years by the claims of the consumerist individualism of dominant political ideology (on both sides of the Atlantic), and exacerbated by recent pressures of economic rationalization in health care (an arena in which technical rather than political processes and solutions currently hold sway; Carr-Hill 1991). Mechanic (1995: 1491) points to the narrow research focus in the US on 'technical and operational issues', and the subsequent neglect of 'patterns of care' in favour of 'alternative financial frameworks'. The considerable usefulness of qualitative data and interpretive methodologies for the informing of practice and policy (not to mention their cost-effectiveness considering the enormous sums already employed in clinical trials) is rarely discussed as part of the quality of life and psychosocial oncology agenda. In failing to look at social context – at *similarities* between patients, treatments, and experiences, and at relationships between elements of the experience of illness and treatment – there is a corresponding failure to develop an informative 'picture' of quality of life, in what it consists, and how it is to be maximized and safeguarded.

We would like to address some key ideas about quality of life of cancer patients in treatment that have emerged from our analysis of the material presented in this book, with reference to some related literature in three broad areas. We will draw attention to areas in which practice and organization could be changed to serve the needs of patients better. In attempting to do this, we are not implying that the content of our book is an adequate basis for the implementation of such changes, but rather that they are implicated within the reported material. Our emphasis in the discussion of this material, both here and elsewhere in this book, is not on the characteristics or efforts of *individual* carers. Rather, we are most concerned with highlighting areas for the improvement of the health care *system*, as it affects cancer patients' experience of treatment.

A definition of 'quality of life'

Most centrally, we have portrayed quality of life as a *social* concept, as residing in relationships between individuals and groups; quality of life consists in the multi-level *connection* of the individual and group, both within local worlds of experience and with the larger social world. The quality of this connection depends in large part on resources, and on the processes by which resources are (differentially) distributed.[1] It is argued here that ideas about resources must be crucial to any conceptualization of quality of life. The resources dealt with most closely in this discussion have been those of time, energy and attention, and a central concern has been the drain of treatment on these for individual patients and their families. Chronic illness and its treatment can be seen as an attack on the resources of time, money, strength, vitality, and the ability to 'pay' (focus) attention, which is an attack on personal identity itself. Mihaly Csikszentmihalyi, in his book *The Evolving Self*, posits attention as the organizer of consciousness:

> Basically, what we can be aware of at any time is limited by our ability to pay attention, which is a limited resource. Attention is the psychic energy that we need to think with, to act with, to remember with . . . The sum of what we attend to over time is *our life* [author's emphasis].
>
> (Csikszentmihalyi 1993: 301)

In a very central sense, quality of life in treatment is about the quality of care and safeguarding those resources most important to it of energy, time and attention. Cancer treatment professionals are concerned with the maximizing of 'lifetime', but need as well to focus on the protection of patients' daily expenditures of time ('life time') and energy, as these directly impact on quality of life.

'Quality of life strategies' within this perspective, then, must be seen to include those that maximize the resources of time and energy for individuals and families. These kinds of strategies can be seen in terms of notions of 'the quality of care', and improved management by agents of patients' treatment and treatment calendars. At a higher level, however, there are issues of resources that go beyond the immediate contexts of health care and involve the wider political arena more specifically: resources like good housing; safe environments; money; leisure and recreation opportunities; employment; good working conditions; freedom of movement and so forth. These are also 'health-related', and facilitate the positive use, augmentation and regeneration of time and energy, all of which greatly affect 'quality of life'.

The notion of 'resource' is a 'middle range' concept, one that 'bridges the gap between what have traditionally been described as the micro and macro levels and, in so doing, helps dissolve what is in reality a false dichotomy' (Gabe and Thorogood 1986: 740). The concept of resource fulfils its bridging function well 'because it contains both structural and experiential dimensions' (1986: 760). In this book, one aim of Chapter 5 was to illustrate how the experiential details of people's resources needs and use (while living and managing the treatment calendar) are related to tensions and problems within the much broader spheres of resources avail-ability and management of particular institutions, the health service itself, and in the social world encompassing the contexts of health care.

In looking at the management *work* of patients and families, resources-related questions about recognition of and reward for labour are high-lighted. There is, however, an important distinction to be drawn between the character of the patient's vs. the physician's work. In positing the view of illness as a political process, Gerson (1976: 219) suggests (as does Friedson, 1970) that the 'organisations of medical situations and medical work' be attended to, and not the individual characteristics of those within medical settings. Gerson sees a fundamental contradiction between the interests of the physician and the patient, in that 'the physician's *work* is the disabling of the patient's *self*', and while the physician must manage both his work and the patient's disease simultaneously, 'the patient must manage his disease *and the physician's work*' (1976: 220, Gerson's italics). In medical situations then,

> The contradictions inherent in the fact that a single organism embodies one person's work and another person's self come rapidly to the fore and generate a host of detailed management problems for both physi-cian and patient. These problems are inherently political.
>
> (1976: 221)

They are also inherently *moral*, in terms of the justification of resources use by both patients and agents in the treatment calendar.

Within the political processes of resources management that characterize medical (and illness) work, 'norms' are produced in the form of constraints and expectations of conduct, and the process by which they are produced is a political one, involving the exercise of power. Gerson remarks:

> One of the most powerful strategies for handling this situation is the ability of the physician (and often nurses as well) to define the prob-lematic conduct of the patient as 'symptomatic' rather than political, and thus react by prescribing rather than negotiating.
>
> (1976: 221)

If, in doing their management work in the treatment calendar, patients' actions challenge or obstruct the biomedical goals of disease management, or the goals of the organization within which this work occurs, they can be, and often are, interpreted in terms of 'deviance'. This 'deviance' has been reconstituted in the psychosocial oncology literature primarily as the failure to 'cope' well, emanating from personality characteristics of the patient. Thus, patients' work is perpetually vulnerable to, and threatened by, disqualification as 'poor coping', dysfunctional behaviour, or unreason-able conduct. This is not generally a risk for the work of professionals, however (although those who fall foul of their more powerful colleagues may have their voices disqualified in similar fashion). Also, even while it can be argued that the management work of professionals and patients in the health care context may not be far apart in substance (the goal of successful management of illness and treatment in enabling better living is a goal common to both professionals and patients, though for different reasons and in different ways), the status of this work differs greatly; professionals are rewarded by power and status for their work, and patients are not. Rather, patients must deal with contexts in which resources are scarce, all the time vulnerable to a deviance focus that could suddenly disqualify their efforts.

Having pointed to these two important issues in the consideration of quality of life as *socially* constituted – resources and power in the management work of both patients and agents in the health care context – we will turn to a discussion of quality of life as it appears in relation to three areas of related research in an effort to draw back from the detail of the book discussion and place the ideas presented in a broader perspective. These three areas include: health economics and quality of life, physicians' management of health care, and social support.

Quality of life assessment in health economics and the new rationality in resources allocation

An obvious arena for the use of 'quality of life' assessment is that of the rationalization of resources in the health care system, and the consumerist ethos of the previous British government. Thirty years ago, there was little input by economists into health care, a situation that is dramatically changed today, with recent advances in economics allowing it to go beyond the analysis of tangible and marketed wealth to analysis of the provision of services in both private and public sectors (Whynes 1992). However, some critics have charged that the apparent move toward rationalization in the allocation of resources (particularly between geographical areas) in the health service is illusory, in that the lack of guiding principles in determining the allocation policy has led to the risk of (flawed) statistical procedures, determining policy 'by default' (Carr-Hill and Sheldon 1992). While there are problems with the methodology used (Carr-Hill and Sheldon point to difficulties with the RAWP – Resources Allocation Working Party – formula and with the Jarman Index upon which the 'deprived area' payment to GPs is based), of greater concern is the lack of clarification of the objectives of expenditures, complicated by the lack of a model for the assessment of variations in need. In the attempt to embrace rationality within the health care system, the statistical cart seems to be pulling the policy horse.

There is some discussion within this debate of the potential for the use of a 'unidimensional' measure of quality of life as an output measure to assess the effectiveness of interventions (by way of assessing satisfaction of need and justifying allocation). The obvious example of this is the QALY, or 'quality adjusted life year'. Carr-Hill (1991: 354) describes the resource 'allocation problem' that the QALY is purported to address (given that allocation is primarily based on the criterion of efficiency) as that of comparing inputs and outputs. He points to the 'ambition' of such an approach to

> generate a complete description of the health effects of a health care program and combine them into a utility function. Despite this broad *ambition*, it is usual to consider only the patient's 'quality of life' and not the effects upon the carers and family of the patient. Moreover, despite the name, it is not claimed to be a global (utility?) measure of the 'quality of life' as that term is commonly understood [cites social indicators of well-being approaches, Andrews and Withey 1976], that is, encompassing happiness or satisfaction with the whole range of life domains. In fact, given the known difficulties of aggregating across individual utility functions, it is more usual to interpret a health index 'as a pseudo-quantity measure of an individual's health rather than as a utility number' [cites Culyer 1978: 89].

Indexes are in *general* (even without the added complication that the multidimensional concept of 'quality of life' brings with it to the problem of measurement) 'suspect', because scores given to scale points are often entirely arbitrary (1991: 355). Carr-Hill is quick to emphasize that the kinds of *data* suggested by the proponents of the QALY should be collected and are valuable (a point made by many commentators in the quality of life field in support for the QALY is that the systematic collection of quality of life data would result from its adoption). However, he points out that there are problems with the adequacy of the database in informing treatment decisions for individuals, and, if adequate data are obtained, how the different elements should be combined.

Also, evaluation is not purely a technical matter, even should the technique be adequate to the practical rigours of the task. Evaluation is shaped by political influences, in the selection of criteria, in the organizational context in which it is carried out, and in the reporting of findings: 'finally, evaluators themselves operate as political actors both within and outside evaluation activities' (Carr-Hill 1991: 359). The restrictions on the QALY are legion, stemming from the fact that it is not a global utility measure, and provides no basis for the comparing of different programmes or policies. Nor can it be used to compare health benefits from expenditure of resources in the health care system with expenditure outside it in generating health (on housing, for example) (1991: 360). In this regard, McTurk (1991: 1601) points out that data can 'gain a life of its own once published in league tables and journals'. He criticizes two studies which used QALY data to make invalid comparisons (costs per QALY were drawn from different sources).

Conversely, Barnett (1991) sees QALYs as an answer to the problem of comparability and definitional confusion in the arena of drug trials research. In this perspective, the selection of which questionnaire to use in assessing treatments is 'a crucial one' (1991: 42c) but only insofar as its content relates to the specific disease, not in terms of its underlying conceptual assumptions. Similarly, van Knippenberg *et al.* (1992) state that choice of quality of life measure depends upon the clinical interests of the decision maker employing them, and the basic choice in quality of life measurement is between either physical indicators of quality of life or psychological/psychiatric ones. While it can be desirable to measure these aspects of treatment experience, it is arguable whether such functional status measurements are of *quality of life*; it is more accurate to state that the measurement is of the 'quality of *functional* living', for example. It is certainly true that that which is to be measured and the uses to which the measurement will be put should guide selection of the measurement tool, but the issue of the relationship of methodology to results should not be reduced to this pragmatic level ('health-related' quality of life seems to relate solely to the particular disease and treatments under consideration, rather than to the broader arena of illness and treatment experience). There can be no facile separation of methodology from research findings: the wording of items, reflecting the conceptual assumptions employed in the measure, has a definite formative impact on the information relayed. Carr-Hill emphasizes a crucial point in this regard, and one that bears much relevance for quality of life assessment outside the health economics field as well as within it: that 'index numbers are not an observation upon the world; they are *generated* and *produced* by a specific set of technical procedures, and the QALY is no exception. In turn, technical procedures are not neutral; they serve different interests, and this should be made explicit' (1991: 361). A more explicit and sophisticated approach to the problem and implications of methodology is needed to inform the discussion of quality of life measurement and its uses.

Because technical assessments are shaped by conceptual frameworks and assumptions that are in turn linked to political agendas, great care must be taken in interpreting the results of quality of life studies, and in the uses to which the concept of 'quality of life', however this is constituted, is put. The vogue for 'rationality' in the health service relates to the previously mentioned 'scientism' so obvious in the realm of quality of life and psychosocial oncology: what must be remembered is that measurement and the development of new technical tools in themselves are not equivalent to political *solutions*, and the use of some definition and measure of quality of life as a means to rationalize resources, champion one treatment over another, or one institution over another is potentially a politically powerful one.

A problem of resource allocation and rationalization in the health service is one of increasing efficiency while not decreasing *access* (D'Ambrosia 1991). A main concern raised by the use of the – variously defined, often overly-restrictive or vague – notion of 'quality of life' in the allocation of health care resources is its potential use to exclude certain individuals from receiving treatment altogether. The definition of the concept of quality of life in any context of use will determine that use (along with other political dimensions of the evaluation context). Dean (1990) points to a US federal government-commissioned study in the early 1980s into the benefits of hospice care vs. conventional (hospital) care of terminally ill patients, that was supposed to assist Congress in making decisions about funding for hospices. The outcome measure used was the Spitzer Quality of Life Index (1981), which assesses performance status. Funding was almost withheld on the basis that researchers were not able to demonstrate significant differences in 'quality of life', as measured using this instrument, between hospice and conventional setting patients. A concern here is that government finance bodies are in a position to adopt a specific definition of quality of life for purposes of resource allocation that could ultimately determine the content of quality of life (Dean 1990).

In Britain, there is a lack of systematic connection between the research arena and political decision making, and government interests are served by choosing which research to use to defend policy positions. Hunter and Pollitt (1992: 164) report that instances of the *systematic* use of results of health services research in Britain to inform government policy 'are so rare as to be almost negligible'. More common is the selective and opportunistic use of research findings to support *existing* policies, or favoured directions in policy making. For example, one small section of Whitehead's *The Health Divide* (Townsend *et al.* 1988), on lifestyles and health, was abstracted from its much broader context of unequal access to conditions that promote health, to support the Conservative government's emphasis on individual responsibility for health. The lack of systematic attention to policy construction means that 'policy' occurs by default: in the US health care rationing occurs 'informally' through differential access, co-payment practices, and differential availability of physicians, while in the UK queuing provides a form of rationing (Rineberg 1991). Pope (1991) has pointed out that the 'queue' is considered to be an entity in government health policy, and not seen as an *account*, a way of describing a situation. In neglecting to recognize the political utility of the quality of life concept and the selectivity with which government-level policy makers deal with health research generally, those who devise measures and carry out assessments of quality of life risk being co-opted into political agendas that may ultimately come to dominate how quality of life is viewed. The replacement of biomedical dominance in the health care arena with economic dominance (Carr-Hill 1991) is not a favourable outcome.

Management in health care

The management ethos of the dominant political ideology in 1990s Britain has pervaded the debate on health care. Improving management is seen as the main means of resolving the alleged crisis in health care systems (Hunter 1991). There is also international interest in the management roles of doctors in different systems of health care at this time, and an increasing participation of doctors in health care management generally, within an environment of scarce resources and increasing costs (Duran-Arenas *et al.* 1991). The Griffiths Report (Griffiths 1983) provides a sort of management manifesto for the assessment and running of health care that has displaced former ideas about 'service and the public good which had hitherto provided the dominant ethos' of the health service (Townsend *et al.* 1988: 24–5). In this management perspective, 'management' is

> about establishing procedures in which activity can be measured against clearly defined objectives. It involves breaking down an activity into inputs and outputs and developing procedures for monitoring the achievement of one against the other. But to do this it becomes essential to be able to measure activity, and in something as complex as health care this cannot be done without ignoring key aspects of treatment and recovery and over-simplifying measures of outcome.

There is a sense in which this type of management ignores the social contexts of health care and of the health care service, which, it is argued here, are crucial to the 'quality of life' of patients. Also, the debate over the management roles of doctors tends to focus on the point of tension between the *clinical* role of the doctor in his or her commitment to management of the individual patient, and the involvement of the doctor in the bureaucratic processes of the larger organization (Duran-Arenas *et al.* 1991; Hunter, 1991, 1992). Focusing the debate at this level, however, suggests that medical management of the individual case is not a problematic health service management issue, whereas the running of the health service itself *is*. This neglects the level of case management, and the considerable problems that can exist within it of consistent and complete treatment calendar management.

Treatment (service) management at the level of the individual patient is not always 'run', overseen, and managed effectively, and those who lose out are patients and their families. Also, the articulation of the management arena in terms of a *dual* role for doctors suggests that management of the individual patient and of the service is somehow separate (we are sure that writers on the subject are unlikely to believe that it is, but this is an implication in setting up the doctor's clinical role as separate from service management). It is doubtful whether 'meso'- and 'macro'-level management strategies (Hunter 1991) will amount to much unless the 'micro' management arena is addressed. For example, absentee consultants may take a toll on the education of medical students and juniors, and this in turn becomes a problem for the service. There is a sense in which clinical management is assumed as implicit within the service, and not as something that needs to be addressed systematically.

In Britain, the Calman-Hine Report (Chief Medical Officers' Expert Advisory Group on Cancer 1995), with its proposed framework of a three-tiered approach to cancer services (primary care, cancer units, and cancer centres), focuses on many of the issues discussed in this book (the work we have presented in this book was completed before the report was released). Since its acceptance by the government, the report has engendered a great deal of discussion in which the need to overcome fragmentation in the provision of cancer services and to reduce the 'lottery factor' governing the quality of care received by patients have been central topics. So far, much has been discussed, but there is little secondary literature to indicate concrete change. Commentators point out that change in terms of improved outcomes for cancer patients is likely to take time to establish, from five to ten and even twenty years for some cancers (Millar 1997). Improvement in communication between professional groups involved in the care and treatment of cancer patients at both primary and secondary care levels, and between these groups and patients, is said to have been an immediate outcome of the report's recommendations. So also has the raising of the profile of cancer within the NHS, and progress has been reported in the movement towards specialization within the district general hospitals to qualify as cancer units (Richards 1997). Primary care and cancer centres remain areas where progress has been less apparent, and there has been reportedly no evidence of analysis of the costs of making the proposed changes (Richards 1997; Sikora 1997). The shortage (or lack of NHS commitment) of funds is cited as a major problem in realizing the aims of the report, as is the continuing shortage of medical and clinical oncologists and specialist nurses whose roles were highlighted by the report (Moore 1997; Sikora 1997).

That care should be patient-centred is a major focus of the report, and the metaphor of the 'cancer journey' seems to have been widely embraced. This image underscores the importance of continuity of care, clear information, choice and guidance through the various stages of treatment within a connected and strategically planned, 'fast-track' service. That coordinated, consistent management of a patient's journey by a range of cooperating professionals is now officially on the agenda as a major contributing factor to success in cancer treatment represents an important step forward. The importance of supportive care for both the patient and family at all stages of the illness is another crucial recognition given voice in the report, and the involvement of palliative care services at earlier stages of the disease will contribute much to realizing such care.

It is the contention of this discussion that clinicians will have to concern themselves with quality of life as a social construct in a real way, in order to address the management needs of patients at the case level, and to take part in health care and service management at organizational levels. This management need not be elaborate: it involves the consistent keeping track of details, and providing a touchstone for patients and families. The management of patients' and families' time and energy is a central 'quality of life' concern for health care, and cannot be divorced from other factors, like response to treatment, functional status and psychological well-being. 'Health-related' quality of life is not a pragmatic solution to the problem of definition in the arena of quality of life when it excludes the social reality of cancer patients (a social reality that includes the treatment centre and hospital, to an increasing extent as disease progresses).

Issues of organizational change can be better understood and addressed by inclusion of clinical management issues. The doctor's role as manager of patients' treatment calendars needs to be problematized, not taken for granted, or kept at the level of doctor–patient interaction. In the accounts of patients interviewed for this study, management of the individual patient seemed at times to be the province, ultimately, of no one. Senior agents often appeared to dip in and out of the case management/treatment calendar management scenario at will, or as the result of accepted practice, such as allowing juniors to handle large amounts and types of work unsupervised. In fact, much of the interactional work of treatment calendar management is delegated to junior and lower status staff. This feature of the clinical context suggests there may be problems with clinicians' knowledge of patients' needs regarding the treatment calendar, and of the patients themselves.

'Empowerment' in relationships can be said to consist in 'the act of giving and receiving, exchanging the basic life commodities of energy and attention' (Baldwin 1991: 287). Empowerment of patients and families within the treatment setting takes place in exchanges between patients and between patients and professionals of these 'basic life commodities' or resources. A central aspect of quality of care that can also be seen as a condition of empowering relationships is *continuity*, which is perhaps most directly experienced (or not) in relationships between key professionals and patients. Cancer is a chronic illness, and patients may be faced throughout treatment by many doctors, without one in particular assuming long-term responsibility, a feature that can produce 'considerable insecurity' (Hietanen 1996). It is through the course of discussions with professionals and other patients that a cancer diagnosis is transformed from crisis event to a condition of life, something that must be lived with.

This kind of 'psychosocial care' of the patient is often viewed as the province of social workers and counsellors (who may or may not be present in adequate numbers in treatment settings). Indeed, these latter groups tend to see psychosocial oncology as being *about* 'supportive care' and survivorship issues, rather than the diagnosis and prescriptive treatment of 'distress'. For those concerned with psychosocial care, helping patients to 'live with' cancer is a more appropriate goal than helping them to 'cope with' it. But more concern for the tasks of living with cancer and its treatment needs to be shown by those professionals who oversee treatment's technical operations and plans. Turner (1995: 39) points out that the doctor–patient relationship is still based on an acute illness model, in which the aim of the medical regimen is to get the ill person back to an active social role. This relationship is therefore temporary, the doctor and patient 'committed to breaking their relationship rather than forming a social connection as a stable and permanent system of interaction'. Within chronic illness, however (and, for that matter, preventive medicine), the doctor–patient relationship is more often long-term, with the patient moving in and out of periods of 'normal' social involvement at home and at work.

One of the benefits of consistent contact with the same professional(s) is the possibility of a more coherent treatment experience for patients and family members. Through consistent contact, 'attention to the trivia of daily treatment and the focus on the technological requirements set the ground for more significant encounters, when difficulties of course and prognosis are addressed' (Del Vecchio Good *et al.* 1994: 857). Mattingly (1994: 814–15), in describing an occupational therapy session in which a therapist 'works to emplot a series of actions . . . weaving them into a meaningful whole', points out the difference between 'treatment as mere sequence, just one medical intervention after another, and treatment as structured narratively, one thing building upon another'. It is against the backdrop of dependable relationships with treatment professionals that meaningful connections between events or sequences of events in the treatment calendar appear. Linked closely to continuity of *contact* with professionals is the notion of coherent treatment calendar *management* of the individual patient, and the centrality of the treatment *plan* in providing a 'chart' of the journey through treatment. Rappaport (1990: 192) underscores the importance of plans (which involve constructions of the future) for meaningful experience by drawing on the metaphor of sailing:

> It is possible to sail a boat, for example, without charts or a compass. However, the absence of a chart prevents the possibility of a journey: one is limited to 'day' sailing, so that new destinations and new challenges are out of reach.

When patients lack consistent contact with professionals who can explain the logic and form of the treatment calendar, they do not experience treatment as a 'journey', or as a 'story', an experience with form, coherence and meaning. Rather, they remain stranded in 'the world of immediacy' of he clinic, where 'endings are rarely made explicit and progression is measured in calibrated bits' (Del Vecchio Good *et al.* 1994: 857).

The current management rhetoric is a part of the initiatives introduced by the previous government in their approach to change in the health service. Consumer needs are seen in both trivial and non-trivial terms, and separating which is which is a difficult task. It is possible, for example, to concentrate on service responsiveness to comparatively trivial 'hotel' aspects, while neglecting more pressing environmental issues like lack of space, or more central service aspects, such as the treatment calendar management prowess of clinicians. However, aspects of the environment of the service that might be deemed 'trivial' might in fact have an enormous impact on the welfare of patients; an attractive environment (comfortable chairs, brightly painted walls, carpets, recessed lighting) is an enormously important aspect of treatment, especially given the amount of time patients spend waiting in clinics. There is a need to guard against tokenism vs. genuine responsiveness in the new concern for consumer satisfaction in health care. The problem perhaps is that 'consumerism' can be too easily invoked (via satisfaction surveys, or 'in-house' poll-taking) to support change, or to overstate the benefits of certain changes in the service, while obscuring real problems with management and response to real need. Aspects of satisfaction with medical care identified by Hall and Dornan (1988) in their review of the satisfaction literature were found to be measured with very uneven frequencies, and the less-studied aspects tended to be 'structural': related to cost, access, bureaucracy and so forth. Only 3 per cent of studies asked about psychosocial concerns. A selective or vague deployment of 'patient satisfaction' (or the more powerful phrase, 'consumer satisfaction') can be a way of preventing real issues of the quality of care from entering the health care arena, while appearing to deal with them.

'Social support' and the quality of life

Levine (1987: 3), in commenting on the 'emergent concern with quality of life' in medical sociology, first points to the success of medical sociology in helping physicians to see that

> decisions to hospitalize, to engage in surgery, or to prolong life through heroic measures do not emanate from a rational, scientific calculus. Instead, they are best viewed as social decisions made by people playing social roles, guided by social values, and located in particular social settings or contexts.

The point has been made earlier in our discussion that quality of life is in danger of being (and has indeed been) co-opted as a tool for, or defence of, an economic rationalism in medicine that strips awareness of social aspects at all levels in health care and illness experience. In this new rationalism, the 'scientific calculus' of which Levine speaks is replaced by that of economics. Levine goes on to describe the emergence of quality of life concerns in the evaluation of health care as 'a major recent development which I believe compels medicine to acknowledge and respond to the over-riding social dimension in health and illness'. He then produces the caveat that health-related quality of life, or that most amenable to medical influence, will have to be constantly distinguished from that which 'resides in the social conditions of our larger world'. Levine fears the 'banalization' of 'quality of life' if the broadness of the term is not qualified in medical sociology. Yet the restriction of quality of life to medically relevant aspects of life leaves medicine (and economics) in control of the definition of the area. It also leads to the stripping away of precisely that social context that medical sociology has worked to include in the medical discourse about treatment and illness (and with which it has attempted to *change* this discourse).

'Social support' is an area of research encompassed by psychosocial oncology and quality of life research, plagued by similar conceptual vagaries, and dominated by a focus on measurement that effectively prohibits exploration of social *context* in illness and treatment. Problems of conceptual clarity remain after years of research in US psychosocial oncology (Kobasa *et al.* 1991), and there is no indication that this situation is different for British research. These authors do however raise the issue of the ignoring of social *environment* in psychosocial research in favour of 'social support'. Social support is 'traditionally' seen in psychosocial oncology as an 'interactional entity involving transactions of emotion, concern, "goods and services", information, and appraisal' (1991: 789); transactions, in other words, of resources. What needs to be pointed out here is that the notion of resources should link the interactional arena of 'social support' with social environment, and that, indeed, it is difficult sensibly to separate 'support' from 'environment'.

In a perspective that sees social support and environment as necessarily interdependent, 'social support' cannot be seen as emanating from the informal sector alone. Williams (1991), in arguing against the individualism of both the (then) 'New Right' governmental focus on personal responsibility and the consumer focus of organizations such as the 'independent living movement' of disabled people, points out that mediation by formal agencies can be welcomed by people who are worried about having to ask their families and close others for more help. The welfare state needs to be seen, he argues, 'not as something upon which people are dependent, but as a resource which can empower people in living autonomously' (1991: 522). Lack of social support for an individual dealing with chronic illness may be a part of a broader group problem of inequalities in health linked to inequalities in conditions of living, the uneven process of the distribution of resources and lack of choice that access to resources bestows on the individual (Gabe and Thorogood 1986; Calnan and Williams 1991; Williams 1991).

Individuals, beliefs about health, and their actual practices in daily living need to be located in a social context in order to be understood. In a study of ideas about health and social class, for example, Calnan and Williams (1991) found that concerns about health did not appear salient in respondents' accounts of daily life, and that when probed for, stated beliefs did not differ significantly between respondents of different social classes. What did appear to differ was the way in which certain resources ('habits' like smoking, and exercise) were used by respondents of different classes and genders. For working-class women, for example, smoking was seen as a means of relaxation, and an adaptive behaviour, in that it enabled them to maintain equilibrium, and, for instance, avoid losing patience with children. Also, the authors found much discrepancy between 'what has been referred to as respondents' rational "public" discourse on the link between health and behaviour', reflecting the formal dictates of the medical profession, governmental health education programmes and media coverage, 'and the "private" or "informal" realm of individual actions which need to be understood within a broader social–economic and cultural context' (1991: 528). Calnan and Williams conclude that health-related behaviour needs to be addressed with attention to constraints existing in the social setting for the modification of individuals' behaviour. In a similar regard, the assessment of 'social support' in oncologic quality of life work needs to examine the capacity for social environment to constrain and enable individuals' 'coping' with illness and treatment.

An important conclusion Kobasa et al. (1991) reach, however, is that the basic structures and processes of cancer health care environments need to be featured in research to deepen understanding of social support and environment, and in this regard to move beyond the individual as the unit of analysis. Social support needs to be seen as a matter for treatment contexts as well as the 'private' lives of patient and family. An expansion of focus also means including 'broad social indicators', like housing, education and income, as well as cross-cultural research (Marshall 1990). Implicated in this regard is the quality of *family* life (Jassak and Knafl 1990), as the individual is often part of a larger immediate unit, who must also deal with the demands of treatment and the treatment calendar, and whose lives will also be affected by the illness. Cancer can be thought of as a 'family disease', and support needs of partners of adult patients need to be more directly addressed (Davis-Ali et al. 1993). Part of the development of a more contextual approach to the area of 'social support' must surely involve a more critical look at methodologies used in psychosocial oncology to answer specific questions, and a taking on board by researchers of other perspectives offered by other disciplines.

Broadhead and Berton (1991) see the role of the physician as that of providing 'social support' through developing 'rapport' with individual patients to facilitate counselling in order to help the patient to 'mobilise' his or her own support resources, and to target patients for referral to other professionals or groups. This view keeps social support as another diagnostic category, to be monitored by the physician, and targeted for intervention when judged inadequate. The 'quality of care' is implicated by these authors as consonant with this provision of 'social support' from the physician. However, apart from ignoring the fact that much support can and does emerge from the social world of the clinic itself, and within professional–patient relationships, this view also glosses over the importance of treatment calendar management in the provision of support by professionals to patients. Keeping details and arrangements straight, keeping appointments personally and not by proxy (particularly important for those who are seen by the patient as 'key professionals' in the treatment calendar), and communicating the nature of the treatment calendar clearly and openly (and often), are all issues of 'support', 'quality of care', and therefore of quality of life for patients.

A major point we wish to make here is that the aspects of treatment that will have the most impact upon the psychosocial realm will often have more to do with, and be more influenced by, aspects of the treatment *calendar* than by either illness or treatment in themselves. In the treatment calendar, existing relationships with others become more heavily depended upon by patients. These relationships are often changed by the new demands made upon them, and the new medical (social) contexts that have to be navigated by both patients and their families. These contexts can be and are sources of much support, however, from other patients, their families, and from medical professionals. The degree of consistency in professionals' and institutional management of the treatment calendar has an enormous impact on psychosocial well-being during treatment. So also does the nature of the environment in which the treatment work of the treatment calendar is performed (in terms of comfort, space and attractiveness, as well as time). Another way of saying this is that the *quality of care* (as evidenced in the processes and contexts of the treatment calendar) emerges as more important for quality of life, at least in the initial treatment for cancer, than either illness or treatment in themselves. The social aspects of the daily, lived experience of treatment have a profound effect upon the psychological and social lives of patients and their families.

The psychosocial literature on social support often refers to the 'support systems' of patients, and uses other terms that suggest that support by families and the community is a formally organized entity. As Graham (1991) points out, 'informal care' (and this term is consonant with the content domain of 'social support' in psychosocial oncology) is not a system, but a *sector*. It is non-institutional, unpaid and largely provided 'through the bonds of kinship' (1991: 508). Lack of research that takes a critical approach to informal care means that 'the process of legislation assumes rather than explores the organisation of care within the home' (1991: 510). The physician's role in the provision of 'support' is depicted largely in terms of helping the ill person to 'deploy' his or her 'social network' in dealing with illness and treatment. As Graham points out, in the informal sector, access to kinship, not needs or rights, determines who gets what care, so it may not be a simple case of getting the ill person to access an existing resource. The larger community plays an important role in treatment and illness calendar management (as evidenced here by patients' accounts of help received from neighbours and friends), but relatives remain by far the biggest resource in the daily management of illness and treatment. Being without a (willing and dependable) spouse or partner, or other close relatives, is a considerable handicap in obtaining support at all levels of the illness experience. Also, the stress and financial burden of caring may threaten and break the very bonds on which it depends (Graham 1991). The real nature of this 'support' or informal caring (the work of caring in its many forms) is not often addressed in the quality of life and psychosocial literature, although there are indications that this is changing (as intimated in the papers discussed above).

Many of the points made in this book can be related usefully to the issue of counselling in oncology. It is important to re-examine counselling, once the social nature of the treatment experience is recognized and its importance for quality of life is understood and accepted. Prescriptive approaches (often referred to as 'problem-focused') may address symptoms, and problems of dysfunction (and these are not trivial concerns by any means), but they do not deal adequately with the social needs of patients and families. Counselling needs to address itself to problems of treatment calendar management (advocacy), resources, companionship, listening, and group involvement, and to problems and concerns *besides* the cancer or its treatment (and it is easy to forget that not all the problems or concerns that cancer patients have are to do with having or being treated for cancer!). Central to any approach to counselling must be the protection of the ill person's *autonomy*, of their ability to act and to maintain a sense of self through the frequently disabling experience of illness and treatment. Such an approach requires a move beyond the pathologizing and individualistic perspective of psychosocial oncology and the biomedical model. Accounts such as those described in this book can contribute to counselling practice by developing contextual pictures of treatment experience.

Conclusion

The philosophical individualism that has dominated psychosocial oncology (and quality of life) work must yield to a more 'social' view of illness and treatment experience, the kind that a qualitative, context-exploring approach can provide. Functional living is not an adequate model for quality of life (while it may be an aspect of this concept), as it excludes concerns about the quality of care, and much that is integral to the 'private' experience of individuals, and to the meaning of personal experience. The notion of 'health-related' quality of life is particularly misleading, as under this rubric only functional living of an overly restrictive and physically-biased kind is dealt with. The use of a plea for pragmatism in quality of life assessment to exclude the social and political dimensions of chronic illness has been evident in oncology, but if the considerable difficulties of living with cancer are to be addressed (as indeed they rarely are in clinical trials of treatment modes), these dimensions must be included (genuinely) on the oncologic agenda. The view of the individual as the unit of analysis must give way to more sophisticated understanding of measurement and methodologic issues, and a consideration of interpretive approaches to aid in developing contextual understanding. The pseudo-broadening of the medical agenda implied in many descriptions of quality of life assessment in oncology needs to be replaced by a genuine consideration of the *patient's* agenda, as constituted in the illness, treatment, personal, and life calendars of patients, as they are connected to the social world through relationships with others, and as they are enabled and constrained by social processes of which they are a part.

Note

1 Gabe and Thorogood (1986: 742) point to Giddens's (1979) conceptualization of resources, not as 'inert materials possessed by individuals, but as part of a process or set of relations'. Also, Giddens distinguishes between resources and power by pointing out that 'power is not a resource in itself; rather, resources are the vehicles of power, they are the media through which power is exercised routinely in social interaction, and structures of domination reproduced' (Gabe and Thorogood 1986: 742, paraphrasing Giddens 1979: 91–2). The authors point out that Giddens's treatment of 'domination' emphasizes the connection of the latter with the 'asymmetric' distribution of resources.

Appendix

Methodological approach and an account of the analysis

Grounded theory is a symbolic interactionist methodological approach, initially described in Glaser and Strauss (1967) and elaborated in Strauss and Corbin (1990). (The following account of the methodology used in both studies is based on that given in Costain Schou and Hewison 1994 and Costain Schou and Hewison forthcoming.) Symbolic interactionism has its roots in the social psychology of William James, C.H. Cooley and W.I. Thomas, but its principal origins are attributed to G.H. Mead's social psychology. Glaser and Strauss's grounded theory lies within the Chicago School interactionist perspective (Herbert Blumer's elaboration of Mead's approach). Blumer (1969) described three postulates of this perspective: that human action toward things is determined by the meaning the things have for them; that meaning arises from interaction between agents in the social world; and that these meanings are handled and modified through processes of interpretation employed by the individual in dealing with the things encountered. Central to this perspective is that it is *social* interaction, and not the isolated individual, that is responsible for meaning generation (Bibbels and Roebuck 1978).

In grounded theory, theory is generated from data, or pre-existing (grounded) theories are elaborated as incoming data are 'meticulously played against them' (Strauss and Corbin 1994: 273) through the signal technique of constant comparison ('the systematic asking of generative and concept-relating questions' about the data, 1994: 275). Theory development is 'substantive' rather than general, and the aim of the constant comparison process is to develop and verify 'hypotheses', defined as 'statements of relationships between concepts' (1994: 274). Theoretical coding results in descriptions of how the 'substantive codes' may relate to each other as hypotheses to be tested. The testing consists of constant comparison of data with 'emerging' conceptual framework, or theory (defined as plausible relationships between concepts and sets of concepts). The criterion of 'fit' – if and how new situations both do and do not fit into the emerging theory – relates to the validity of the theory, but theories and their validity are fluid, affected by the passage of time and new conditions. They are interpretations, and as such must be elaborated and qualified (Strauss and Corbin 1994).

The interpretation of patients' accounts presented in the pages of this book is not intended to stand as the only possible account, or as the 'truth' retrieved from 'data'. Research stories like this one do not 'emerge' (though that term is used often in accounts of grounded theory and other interpretive approaches) from data. Rather, they are constructed through the grounded analysis of *text*. The goal of the analysis is to include meaningfully (deal with, recognize) all the interview material analysed (including 'negative cases' and dissenting voices) in order to attend to each participant's personal narrative while constructing a context in which to locate it. This is quite different from the lists of themes and topics produced in content analysis.

Below is a description of how we came to use this method during our first study. A central concern of ours was to treat the interview transcriptions as text and discourse produced in a very specific situation (the interview), an interaction between the interviewer (KCS) and the respondent (and, in most cases, the respondent's spouse or partner as well). We wished not to lose sight of the specific constitutive features of this situation, the different ways in which respondents might be presenting themselves to the interviewer, and the interviewer's effect upon and contribution to the discourse produced. This is not to mean we were preoccupied with 'bias', but rather with the interview as a specific situation involving several participants engaged in constructing the story of 'treatment experiences' which was our focus. In the book, we have tried to give an account of the different discourses produced in these interviews, as well as producing a story of treatment experience to which all the respondents' voices can be heard to contribute.

Data collection method

In the two parts of the study, several one- to three-hour interviews were conducted with cancer patients being treated with radiation alone or with radiotherapy and chemotherapy. Most patients had had some surgery before beginning adjuvant therapy. The interviews were semi-structured (initially based on information drawn from the literature, but adapted through the course of interviewing to reflect new information from our respondents, as well as that from the observation time KCS spent each week in the treatment centre prescription and review clinics). The respondents were contacted at prescription clinic, held on the Monday of each week, and introduced to the study through a brief contact meeting with KCS during which they were also given written information. Those who agreed to participate were then contacted by telephone to arrange a convenient time to be interviewed in their homes. Respondents were interviewed once, midway through their main treatment schedule, for the first part of the study, and two to four times at specific points during post-surgical treatment for the second. Before the first interview in both phases, respondents had filled out two questionnaires on their own at home (the Ontario Cancer Institute Scale, Selby *et al.* 1984, and the MacAdam Quality of Life Questionnaire, MacAdam and Smith 1987). All the interviews were transcribed in full.

Starting point for the analysis: theme analysis

Because the first part of the study was an introductory one for us into the area of 'quality of life' and cancer treatment, we did not want inadvertently to overlook any detail in the transcripts. We began the analysis during data collection in order to inform the interviewing process. In selecting a method for subsequent analysis we had two main concerns:

1 We wished to account for all the data while operating with as few analytic assumptions as possible. We wished to focus on patterns of meaning and interpretation presented in respondents' accounts without presuming what these might be beforehand.

2 We were concerned with preserving the interviews' essential features as *discourse* (Mishler 1986) and with using the accounts and language of respondents as the *objects* of analysis, not just as an analytic resource (Potter and Wetherell 1987). We were concerned to maintain a discursive focus in the analysis of these accounts rather than speculate on cognitive structures, motivations, etc. because the analysis was to be of interview transcripts and notes, not of *people per se*.

We set out to do a generic 'theme' analysis (although in the course of interviewing and transcription, which had taken place alongside one another, preliminary analysis in the form of close reading of transcripts had shaped the questioning in subsequent interviews throughout the course of the interviewing). The purpose of this 'atheoretical' analysis was to *develop* ideas from a critical reading of the data, rather than to impose a conceptual framework upon it. Earlier, in summarizing the item content of the OCI and MacAdam questionnaires, we had identified several broad content domains: physical and psychological functioning, psychosocial concerns, information and treatment. We had initially tried to represent these four domains in the questions included in the interview so as to allow for a comparison with the questionnaire results. These four headings appeared to encompass the content domain of cancer patients' 'quality of life' as defined in the literature.

We decided to order the data into these four content domains before proceeding with further analysis. This enabled us to divide the data into manageable groups, and to reread the interview transcripts as a group. We divided the interview transcripts into excerpts, ensuring that each excerpt retained as much context as possible (including interviewer's questions and comments), and then assigned them to one of the four content domains. All excerpts were labelled so that they could be traced back to their place in the transcript.

We included a fifth heading to encompass the rest of the data – diagnosis experiences – as all the interviews featured narrative accounts of the process of becoming diagnosed. It appeared that 'treatment' was described as beginning *before* the diagnosis was reached, from the first presentation with symptoms or first screening. The diagnosis narratives covered this pre-operative/extended diagnosis stage, whereas our actual interview *questions* had initially focused on the post-operative treatment stage. The assumption that 'treatment' was confined to a schedule or set of schedules following diagnosis did not seem accurate, as respondents described 'the whole thing' as beginning with a first consultation pre-diagnosis, and as more or less continuous from that point (discontinuities, such as poor communication between diagnostic setting and the treatment centre, were noted in great detail by respondents).

Once all the data excerpts had been read and grouped into the content domains, the process of thematic coding was begun. In order to accomplish the identification of themes in the interview transcript excerpts, we used two procedures:

1 A line-by-line analysis of individual excerpts within each content category. Each discrete event, process, perspective, description and so forth described in an excerpt was labelled. These labels were intended to describe content in a more *conceptual* way than the four content domains: each label had to both refer to a phenomenon being constructed in an account and also provide a building-block for a more dimensional grouping, like a *theme*, within which many similar accounts would be grouped.
2 The constant comparison of excerpts, first within each content category and then, as the analysis proceeded, across content domains. During this constant comparison, similarities and differences between both excerpts (discrete accounts) *and* the conceptual labels we devised to describe them were noted, and these conceptual labels were grouped thematically.

As thematic groupings became more detailed (as more and more sub-themes were identified for each grouping), they began to cover a broader dimensional range (as more properties of described context, aspects of context, experiences etc. were coded) and each excerpt had to be located within any particular grouping according to where it *fitted* within this range (not merely slotted in under a single, broad heading). Groupings changed and multiplied as we sought to locate all the excerpts. We were interested in locating each excerpt meaningfully within these groupings (thus developing the groupings into categories). We then compared groupings with one another, and worked to delineate relationships between them. The original groupings were no longer *real* in the sense that the emerging thematic framework had transcended them.

Moving from a 'checklist' to a theoretical framework

Towards the end of the analysis, and after having read Glaser and Strauss's *The Discovery of Grounded Theory* (1967), we realized that we had taken steps beyond our initial goal of providing a list of themes. In questionnaire development in the study of quality of life, interview transcripts are analysed to produce 'checklists' of items to be further reduced into content domains which are then 'tapped' by items on the resulting QL measure. This process strips context and meaning from interview data. It also ignores such 'data' as discourse, treating it instead as a route to an underlying real and fixed situation. Through both being engaged in and reading about grounded theory techniques, we had the goal of moving beyond an initial list of themes and sub-themes (the checklist approach) toward a more conceptual and integrated understanding of respondents' discourse about treatment experience.

At this stage, the original analysis had been refined: each thematic grouping had become a classification of concepts (a category) focused on a central phenomenon, and contained sub-categories that were: (a) related to each other, and (b) related to a central phenomenon, or category, in various ways.

We also had a *core category* (or central discourse) to which all the others were related which we called *treatment as social interaction*. We had gone from initially viewing the treatment process as neutral, and from focusing on respondents' accounts of their feelings about the *fact* of the cancer, to a deeper view of the construction of treatment in the interview as a social process, one constructed by professionals and patients as individuals in a variety of contexts.

Strauss and Corbin (1990) describe sub-categories related to each category in terms of *causal conditions*, or those that give rise to the phenomenon (or category), and *contextual conditions*, or properties of the category that form the dimensional range of each category. These conditions are the conditions within which *action/interactional strategies* are taken. *Intervening conditions* are broader structural conditions that either facilitate or constrain strategies undertaken. *Action/interactional strategies* themselves are those taken to manage the phenomenon, carry it out, or respond to it. *Consequences* are the results of *strategies* undertaken – the results of *action* or of *interaction*.

In attempting to link sub-categories to their categories, and all main categories to the *core category* in this way, the researcher aims towards theory and away from pure description (Charmaz 1990). A theoretical framework is attempted rather than stopping the analysis at the level of a checklist of themes. This framework should develop to account for all the data, and for as much relationship between interview excerpts and the conceptual labels used to define them as possible.

There is an obvious tension between the realist language of grounded theory method (procedures are aimed at charting 'processes' and 'structures' going on 'out there' in the world as accessed through language and the reports of respondents) and our avowed focus on discourse and constructions of experience in the interview situation. We cannot pretend to have resolved these tensions in our own work (or in the reporting of our work here and in the pages of this book). We view our 'themes' and eventual 'categories' as constructions based on our close reading of both *what* respondents have said and *how* they have said it, not as labels affixed to a static external reality. Our use of the word 'description' is not intended to imply that we regard our respondents' accounts as mere references to such a reality. Rather, we see the content and form of 'descriptions' as constructive of (as constructing) lived experience, at both the personal and social levels. The task of producing descriptions/constructions of experience is one demanded by the interview situation, yet it also seems to be demanded by 'experience' itself. In order to be an 'experiencer', one must be a 'self-storier'. Such 'self-stories' are drawn from, and contribute to, ever-changing societal stories that in turn facilitate and constrain possible future stories, including those of research.

Category example: the expanding social context

Contrary to work stressing the stigma of cancer and the subsequent narrowing of the cancer patient's social world (MacDonald 1988; Fallowfield 1990; Fallowfield and Clark 1991), interview accounts presented a picture of broadened perspective regarding cancer and 'cancer patients'. People identified themselves discursively as members of a wider social context as people with cancer, and as more meaningfully connected with old contexts, as they described the response to their illness from the community. This 'broadening' discourse appeared to arise ultimately out of what we came to see as the struggle for definition that characterized discourse about treatment, and that was facilitated by the production of accounts of treatment experience in interview. *The expanding social context* was an important consequence of all the other categories: respondents described a pervasive broadening of social context which they linked to the community and to their contact with the treatment centre.

The expanding social context

Causal conditions

The essential causal condition was contact – with professionals and other patients, in new medical contexts. This contact was identified by respondents as forced upon them by circumstances/unavoidable, incidental, but also as voluntary or sought-after (respondents as a group described experiencing these aspects of contact in medical contexts). Contact with others was cast as an inescapable fact of treatment brought about initially by the disruption of the 'ordinary' by the 'extraordinary' (the illness) and by the diagnosis process.

Contact

Individual accounts are located at different places within dimensional ranges such as:

- Accounts of the extent or pervasiveness of the expansion of social context.
- When the process started and when it finished (time span and places in treatment trajectory). What starts as an inevitable consequence of illness and diagnosis (the expansion of contexts for experience) can become a more voluntary process of continuing to expand definitions of social context.
- The identified contributions (what kind and how much) of the agents involved, the number of agents and who these are, and the number of settings in which agents are encountered.

Intervening conditions

The amount and type of treatment: chemotherapy patients not receiving radiotherapy can be relatively isolated during treatment, attending clinic much less frequently, and often as outpatients in small hospital clinics rather than large treatment centres. Also, patients having combined schedules may experience more than one treatment setting (a general hospital and specialist treatment centre) and many different types of professional.

Travelling to and from the treatment centre(s): patients without private transport usually use the ambulance service, meaning that their treatment day can last between five and nine hours, depending on how far away they live and how busy the route. Spending this much time on transport was linked in accounts to developing relationships with the same ambulance drivers and the same small group of other patients. Respondents also described becoming aware of the *geography* of treatment – detailing their awareness that other people living near them and far afield were having the same treatment for cancer. The 'space' occupied by the illness in terms of the wider community emerged vividly in respondents' accounts of this apparent shift in perspective.

If the daily routine is maintained: people who described retaining close contact with work or leisure groups and so forth during treatment linked this in interview with finding out about a wider experience with cancer/ chronic illness and treatment than they had known existed. Conversely, two men described using the daily routine of work to 'screen out' the treatment experience and to 'behave as normal'. They described keeping treatment slotted into an existing schedule.

In many ways, treatment at the clinic appeared to flout the very precise boundaries that most people described having in terms of what kinds of conversations to have with whom. Patients who were accompanied to treatment by neighbours and casual acquaintances described forming much closer friendships with these people, even though they had known each other for years previously. Most patients who lived outside City A, in or nearer City B, described living in communities that were less 'friendly' or more anonymous than the 'warmer' City A community. Contact with patients and their families at the City A treatment centre was constructed as supportive and a counterbalance to this anonymity. Patients described sometimes feeling invaded by the reality of the new treatment context of which they were a part, however: for example, the sight of the ambulance arriving every day to collect some patients made the 'extraordinary' public, and part of 'other people's business' in the community.

Action/interaction strategies

Observing: not exactly depicted as a strategy but discursively constructed in interview accounts as an activity that became strategic as time went on. Patients described initially noticing how many gestures of support they received from the community (like cards and phone calls) and how they had identified this as surprising evidence of their connection with this community. There was a voiced sense of surprise at 'how many people cared'.

Constant comparison: respondents described and engaged in constant comparison of themselves with other patients (something they had been expressly – and heavily – warned against doing by clinic staff) and gave voice to the range of others' experiences with the 'same' disease or set of diseases with which they had not been familiar prior to the diagnosis. This appeared in accounts to have contributed to a more dimensional view of the illness and of other people with the illness and to have enabled them to construct and locate themselves within a context they had initially lacked.

Self-disclosure: patients described using the waiting room as a safe place to disclose, and many who described themselves as very 'private' said they were able to disclose details of their illnesses at the treatment centre in informal conversations. Such conversations were vividly recalled in the interviews, and together constructed a view of the centre as a social world.

Consequences

Accounts of expansions in context, experience and meaning were voiced in a context of the struggle to place a highly altered daily life in a more 'ordinary' and 'normal' light. The exposure people described having to a broadened context in which they had had to interact with other people in new ways seemed to have provided them with a source of meaningful new definitions for what they were experiencing and for who they were as members of a group – 'cancer patients'. Interview accounts, rather than dominated by a discourse of 'control' (of self, of life circumstances, etc.) such as that found in the psychosocial oncology literature, seemed focused rather on the need to *define* self and experience, to make it meaningful. In addition to new definitions, old notions of 'normalcy' and 'ordinariness' were applied to the new territory of cancer treatment and illness. This allowed for the discursive location of self in an ambiguous and rapidly changing terrain.

References

Aaronson, N.K., Bullenger, M. and Ahmedzai, S. (1988) A modular approach to quality of life assessment in cancer clinical trials, in *Recent Results in Cancer Research, III*. Heidelberg: Springer-Verlag.

Aaronson, N.K., Meyerowitz, B.E., Bard, M., Bloom, J.R., Fawzy, F.I., Feldstein, M. *et al.* (1991) Quality of life research in oncology: past achievements and future priorities. *Cancer*, 67 (3 Suppl.): 839–43.

Admi, H. (1996) Growing up with a chronic condition: a model of an ordinary lifestyle. *Qualitative Health Research*, 6(2): 163–83.

Anderson, J.M., Blue, C. and Lau, A. (1991) Women's perspectives on chronic illness: ethnicity, ideology and restructuring life. *Social Science and Medicine*, 33(2): 101–13.

Andrews, F. and Withey, S.B. (1976) *Social Indicators of Well Being*. New York: Plenum Press.

Arney, W.R. and Bergen, B.J. (1984) *Medicine and the Management of Living: Taming the Last Great Wild Beast*. Chicago: University of Chicago Press.

Auchincloss, S.S. (1995) After treatment: psychosocial issues in gynecologic cancer survivorship. *Cancer*, Supplement, 76(10): 2117–24.

Baldwin, C. (1991) *Life's Companion: Journal Writing as a Spiritual Quest*. New York: Bantam.

Barnett, D.B. (1991) Assessment of quality of life. *American Journal of Cardiology*, 67(12): 41c–44c.

Beckmann, J.H. (1989) *Breast Cancer and Psyche: A Comparative Psychological Measurement of the Correlates of Breast Cancer*. Odeuse: IDEAS International.

Bibbels, R. and Roebuck, J.B. (1978) The meditation movement: symbolic interactionism and synchronicity, in N.K. Denzin (ed.) *Symbolic Interaction: An Annual Compilation of Research*, Vol. 1: 205–40. Greenwich, CT: JAI Press Inc.

Blanchard, C.G., Labrecque, M.S., Ruckaeschel, J.C. and Blanchard, E.B. (1990) Physician behaviors, patient perceptions and patient characteristics as predictors of satisfaction of hospitalised adult cancer patients. *Cancer*, 65: 186–92.

Bloch, S. and Kissane, D.W. (1995) Psychosocial care and breast cancer. *Lancet*, 346: 1114–15.

Bloom, J.R. (1991) Quality of life after cancer: a policy perspective. *Cancer*, 67 (3 Suppl.): 855–9.

Bloom, J.R., Kessler, L.G. and Pee, D. (1992) Psychosocial assessment of the recovery from mastectomy: a comparison of static and dynamic modeling. *Psychology and Health*, 7(2): 131–46.

Blumer, H. (1969) *Symbolic Interactionism: Perspective and Method*. Englewood-Cliffs: Prentice-Hall Inc.

Bowling, A. (1997) *Measuring Health: A Review of Quality of Life Measurement Scales*, 2nd edn. Buckingham: Open University Press.

Breetvelt, I.S. and van Dam, F.S.A.M. (1991) Underreporting by cancer patients: the case of response-shift. *Social Science and Medicine*, 32(9): 981–7.

Britten, N. (1991) Hospital consultants' views of their patients. *Sociology of Health and Illness*, 13(1): 83–97.

Broadhead, W.H. and Berton, H.K. (1991) Social support and the cancer patient: implications for future research and clinical care. *Cancer*, 67(3 Suppl.): 794–9.

Burish, T.G. (1991) Progress in psychosocial and behavioral cancer research: the need for enabling strategies. *Cancer*, 67 (3 Suppl.): 860–4.

Bury, M. (1991) The sociology of chronic illness: a review of research and prospects, *Sociology of Health and Illness*, 13(4): 451–68.

Calnan, M. and Williams, S. (1991) Style of life and the salience of health: an exploratory study of health-related practices in households from differing socio-economic circumstances. *Sociology of Health and Illness*, 13(4): 506–29.

Carr-Hill, R.A. (1991) Allocating resources to health care: is the QALY (quality adjusted life year) a technical solution to a political problem? *International Journal of Health Services*, 21(2): 351–63.

Carr-Hill, R.A. (1992) The measurement of patient satisfaction. *Journal of Public Health Medicine*, 14(3): 236–49.

Carr-Hill, R.A. and Sheldon, T. (1992) Rationality and the use of formulas in the allocation of resources in health care. *Journal of Public Health Medicine*, 14(2): 117–26.

Cassileth, B.R., Lusk, E., Brown, L., Cross, P., Walsh, W. and Hurwitz, S. (1986) Factors associated with psychological distress in cancer patients. *Medical and Pediatric Oncology*, 14: 251–4.

Charmaz, K. (1983) Loss of self: a fundamental form of suffering in the chronically ill. *Sociology of Health and Illness*, 5: 168–95.

Charmaz, K. (1990) 'Discovering' chronic illness: using grounded theory. *Social Science and Medicine*, 30(11): 1161–72.

Chaturvedi, S.K. (1991) Research note: what's important for quality of life to Indians – in relation to cancer. *Social Science and Medicine*, 33(1): 91–4.

Chief Medical Officers' Expert Advisory Group on Cancer (1995) *A Policy Framework for Commissioning Cancer Services* (the Calman-Hine Report). London: Department of Health.

Clark, J.A., Potter, D.A. and McKinlay, J.B. (1991) Bringing social structure back into clinical decision-making. *Social Science and Medicine*, 32(8): 853–66.

Conrad, P. (1990) Qualitative research on chronic illness: a commentary on method and conceptual development. *Social Science and Medicine*, 30(11): 1257–63.

Corbin, J. and Strauss, A.L. (1988) *Unending Work and Care: Managing Chronic Illness at Home*. San Francisco: Jossey-Bass.

Corney, R., Everett, H., Howells, A. and Crowther, M. (1992) The care of patients undergoing surgery for gynaecological cancer: the need for information, emotional support and counselling. *Journal of Advanced Nursing*, 17: 667–71.

Costain Schou, K. (1993) Awareness contexts and the construction of dying in the cancer treatment setting: 'micro' and 'macro' levels in narrative analysis, in D. Clark (ed.) *The Sociology of Death*. Oxford: Blackwell.

Costain Schou, K. and Hewison, J. (1994) Issues of interpretive methodology: the utility and scope of grounded theory in contextual research. *Human Systems*, 5: 45–68.

Costain Schou, K. and Hewison, J. (forthcoming) Social psychology and discourse: personal accounts as social texts in grounded theory. *Journal of Health Psychology*.

Cox, D.R. (1991) Health service management – a sociological view: Griffiths and the non-negotiated order of the hospital, in J. Gabe, M. Calnan and M. Bury (eds) *The Sociology of the Health Service*. London: Routledge.

Cox, D.R., Fitzpatrick, R., Fletcher, A.E., Gore, S.M., Spiegelhalter, D.J. and Jones, D.R. (1992) Quality of life assessment: can we keep it simple? *Journal of the Royal Statistical Society*, 155: 353–93.

Csikszentmihalyi, M. (1993) *The Evolving Self: A Psychology for the Third Millennium*. New York: HarperCollins.

Cull, A. (1990) Invited review: psychological aspects of cancer and chemotherapy. *Journal of Psychosomatic Research*, 34(2): 129–40.

Culyer, A.J. (1978) *Measuring Health: Lessons from Ontario*. Toronto: University of Toronto Press.

Cunningham, A.J. (1986) Information and health in the many levels of man: toward a more comprehensive theory of health and disease. *Advances*, 1(1): 32–45.

D'Ambrosia, R. (1991) Editorial: Alternatives to rationing health care. *Orthopedics*, 14(7): 747.

Davenport, S., Goldberg, D. and Millar, T. (1987) How psychiatric disorders are missed during medical consultations, *Lancet*, 2: 439.

Davis-Ali, S.H., Chesler, M.A. and Chesney, B.K. (1993) Recognizing cancer as a family disease: worries and support reported by patients and spouses. *Social Work in Health Care*, 19(2): 45–65.

Dean, H.E. (1990) Political and ethical implications of using quality of life as an outcome measure. *Seminars in Oncology Nursing*, 6(4): 303–8.

Deeny, P. and McCrea, H. (1991) Stoma care: the patient's perspective. *Journal of Advanced Nursing*, 16: 39–46.

de Haes, J.C.J.M. and van Knippenberg, F.C.E. (1985) The quality of life of cancer patients: a review of the literature. *Social Science and Medicine*, 20(8): 809–17.

Del Vecchio Good, M., Tseunetsugu, M., Kobayashi, Y., Mattingly, C. and Good, B.J. (1994) Oncology and narrative time. *Social Science and Medicine*, 38(6): 855–62.

Derogatis, L.R., Morrow, G.R., Fetting, J., Penman, D., Piatsetsky, S., Schmale, A.M., Henrichs, M. and Carnicke, C.L. (1983) The prevalence of psychiatric disorders among cancer patients. *Journal of the American Medical Association*, 249: 751–7.

Deyo, R.A. (1991) Editorial: the quality of life, research and care. *Annals of Internal Medicine*, 114(8): 695–6.

Donovan, K., Sanson-Fisher, R.W. and Redman, S. (1989) Measuring quality of life in cancer patients. *Journal of Clinical Oncology*, 7(7): 959–68.

Dreher, H. (1987) Cancer and the mind: current concepts in psycho-oncology. *Advances*, 4(3): 27–43.

Duran-Arenas, L., Asfura, M.B. and Mora, J.F. (1991) The role of doctors as health care managers: an interactional perspective. *Social Science and Medicine*, 35(4): 549–55.

Elston, M. (1991) The politics of professional power: medicine in a changing health service, in J. Gabe, M. Calnan and M. Bury (eds) *The Sociology of the Health Service*. London: Routledge.

Engel, G. (1977) The need for a new medical model: a challenge for biomedicine. *Science*, 196: 129–36.

Ezzy, D. (1993) Unemployment and mental health: a critical review. *Social Science and Medicine*, 37(1): 41–52.

Faden, R. and LePlege, A. (1992) Assessing quality of life: moral implications for clinical practice. *Medical Care*, 30(5 Suppl.): MS166–MS175.

Fakhoury, N., McCarthy, M. and Addington-Hall, J. (1996) Determinants of informal caregivers' satisfaction with services for dying cancer patients. *Social Science and Medicine*, 42(5): 721–31.

Fallowfield, L. (1988) Counselling for patients with cancer. *British Medical Journal*, 297: 727–8.

Fallowfield, L. (1990) *The Quality of Life: The Missing Measurement in Health Care*. London: Souvenir Press.

Fallowfield, L. (1995) Psychosocial interventions in cancer. *British Medical Journal*, 311: 1316–17.

Fallowfield, L. and Clark, A. (1991) *Breast Cancer*. The Experience of Illness Series. London: Tavistock/Routledge.

Fife, B.L. (1994) The conceptualization of meaning in illness. *Social Science and Medicine*, 38(2): 309–16.

Fife, B.L. (1995) The measurement of meaning in illness. *Social Science and Medicine*, 40(8): 1021–8.

Fobair, P. and Mages, N. (1981) Psychosocial morbidity among cancer patient survivors, in P. Ahmed (ed.) *Living and Dying With Cancer*. New York: Elsevier North Holland Inc.

Ford, S., Fallowfield, L. and Lewis, S. (1996) Doctor–patient interactions in oncology. *Social Science and Medicine*, 42(11): 1511–19.

Friedson, E. (1970) *Profession of Medicine: A Study of the Sociology of Applied Knowledge*. New York: Harper and Row.

Gabe, J. and Thorogood, N. (1986) Prescribed drug use and the management of everyday life: the experiences of black and white working-class women. *Sociological Review*, 34(4): 738–72.

Gerhardt, U. (1990) Introductory essay: qualitative research on chronic illness: the issue and the story. *Social Science and Medicine*, 30(11): 1149–59.

Gerson, E.M. (1976) The social character of illness: deviance or politics? *Social Science and Medicine*, 10: 219–24.

Giddens, A. (1979) *Central Problems in Social Theory*. London: Macmillan.

Glaser, B.G. and Strauss, A.L. (1965) *Awareness of Dying*. London: Weidenfeld and Nicolson.

Glaser, B.G. and Strauss, A.L. (1967) *The Discovery of Grounded Theory: Strategies for Qualitative Research*. New York: Aldine De Gruyter.

Gotay, C.C. (1991) Accrual to cancer clinical trials, *Social Science and Medicine*, 33(5): 569–77.

Graham, H. (1991) The informal sector of welfare: a crisis in caring? *Social Science and Medicine*, 32(4): 507–15.

Greer, S. (1987) Introduction to special issue on psychosocial oncology. *Cancer Surveys*, 6(3): 401–2.

Greer, S. and Morris, T. (1975) Psychological attributes of women who develop breast cancer: a controlled study. *Journal of Psychosomatic Research*, 19: 147–53.

Greer, S., Moorey, S. and Watson, M. (1989) Patients' adjustment to cancer: the mental adjustment to cancer (MAC) scale vs clinical ratings. *Journal of Psychosomatic Research*, 33(3): 373–7.

Greer, S., Moorey, S., Baruch, J., Watson, M., Robertson, B., Mason, A. *et al.* (1992) Adjuvant psychological therapy for patients with cancer: a prospective randomised trial. *British Medical Journal*, 304: 675–80.

Griffiths, R. (1983) *NHS Management Inquiry DA (83)38*. London: DHSS.

Guex, P. (1994) *An Introduction to Psycho-Oncology*. London: Routledge.

Hall, J.A. and Dornan, M.C. (1988) What patients like about their medical care and how often they are asked: a metanalysis of the satisfaction literature. *Social Science and Medicine*, 27(9): 935–9.

Hietanen, P.S. (1996) Measurement and practical aspects of quality of life in breast cancer. *ACTA Oncologica*, 35(1): 39–42.

Holland, J.C. (1992a) Psycho-oncology: overview, obstacles and opportunities. *Psycho-Oncology*, 1: 1–13.

Holland, J.C. (1992b) Psycho-oncology: where are we and where are we going? *Journal of Psychosocial Oncology*, 10(2): 103–12.

Hopwood, P. (1992) Progress, problems and priorities in quality of life research. *European Journal of Cancer*, 28a: 1748–52.

Hopwood, P. (1996) Quality of life assessment in chemotherapy trials for non-small cell lung cancer. Are theory and practice significantly different? *Seminars in Oncology*, 23(5) (Suppl. 10): 60–4.

Hopwood, P. and Maguire, P. (1988) Body image problems in cancer patients. *British Journal of Psychiatry*, 153 (2 Suppl.): 47–50.

Hopwood, P., Howell, A. and Maguire, P. (1991a) Psychiatric morbidity in patients with advanced cancer of the breast: prevalence measured by two self-rating questionnaires. *British Journal of Cancer*, 64: 349–52.

Hopwood, P., Howell, A. and Maguire, P. (1991b) Screening for psychiatric morbidity in patients with advanced cancer of the breast: validation of two self-report questionnaires. *British Journal of Cancer*, 64: 353–6.

Horwich, A. and Duchesne, G. (1988) The role of radiotherapy, in R. Tiffany and P. Pritchard (eds) *Oncology for Nurses and Health Care Professionals*, 2nd edn., Vol. 1. London: Harper and Row.

Hunter, D.J. (1991) Managing medicine: a response to the 'crisis'. *Social Science and Medicine*, 32(4): 441–8.

Hunter, D.J. (1992) Doctors as managers: poachers turned gamekeepers? *Social Science and Medicine*, 35(4): 557–66.

Hunter, D.J. and Pollitt, C. (1992) Development in health services research: perspectives from Britain and the United States. *Journal of Public Health Medicine*, 14(2): 164–8.

Illich, I. (1976) *Medical Nemesis: The Expropriation of Health*. New York: Random House.

Jassak, P.F. and Knafl, K.A. (1990) Quality of family life: exploration of a concept. *Seminars in Oncology Nursing*, 6(4): 298–302.

Jenkins, C.D., Jono, R.T., Stanton, B. and Stroup-Benham, C.A. (1990) The measurement of health-related quality of life: major dimensions identified by factor analysis. *Social Science and Medicine*, 31(8): 925–31.

Jenney, M.E.M. (1996) Editorial: Health-related quality of life, cancer and health care. *European Journal of Cancer*, 32A(8): 1281–2.

Jobling, R. (1988) The experience of psoriasis under treatment, in R. Anderson and M. Bury (eds) *Living With Chronic Illness: The Experience of Patients and Their Families*. London: Unwin Hyman.

Jones, D.R., Fayers, P.M. and Simons, J. (1987) Measuring and analyzing quality of life in cancer clinical trials: a review, in N.K. Aaronson and J. Beckmann (eds) *The Quality of Life of Cancer Patients*. New York: Raven Press.

Joyce, C.R.B. (1988) Quality of life: the state of the art in clinical assessment, in S.R. Walker and R.M. Rosser (eds) *Quality of Life: Assessment and Application*. London: MTP Press.

Kleinman, A. (1992) Local worlds of suffering: an interpersonal focus for ethnographies of illness experience. *Qualitative Health Research*, 2(2): 127–34.

Knudtson, P. and Suzuki, D. (1992) *Wisdom of the Elders*. Toronto: Stoddart Publishing Co.

Kobasa, S.C.O., Spinetta, J.J., Cohen, J., Crano, W.D., Hatchett, S., Kaplan, B.H. et al. (1991) Social environment and social support. *Cancer*, 67 (3 Suppl.): 788–93.

Levanthal, H., Nerenz, D.R. and Levanthal, E. (1982) Feelings of threat and private views of illness: factors in dehumanization in the medical care system, in A. Baum and J.E. Singer (eds) *Advances in Environmental Psychology, Vol. 4: Environment and Health*. New Jersey: Lawrence Erlbaum Assoc.

Levine, S. (1987) The changing terrains in medical sociology: emergent concerns with quality of life. *Journal of Health and Social Behaviour*, 28: 1–6.

Levine, S. and Kozloff, M.A. (1978) The sick role: assessment and overview. *Annual Reviews of Sociology*, 4: 317–43.

Liang, L.P., Dunn, S.M., Gornan, A. and Stuart-Harris, R. (1990) (personal correspondence) 'Identifying priorities of psychosocial need in cancer patients'.

MacAdam, D.B. and Smith, M. (1987) An initial assessment of suffering in terminal illness. *Palliative Medicine*, 1: 37–47.

MacDonald, L. (1988) The experience of stigma: living with rectal cancer, in L. Anderson and M. Bury (eds) *Living With Chronic Illness*. London: Unwin Hyman.

MacDowell, I. and Newell, C. (1987) *Measuring Health: A Guide to Rating Scales and Questionnaires*. Oxford: Oxford University Press.

McIntosh, J. (1974) Processes of communication, information seeking and control associated with cancer: a selective review of the literature. *Social Science and Medicine*, 8: 167–87.

McTurk, L. (1991) A methodological quibble about QALYs. *British Medical Journal*, 302(6792): 1601.

Maguire, P. and Selby, P. (1989) Assessing quality of life in cancer patients. *British Journal of Cancer*, 60: 437–40.

Marshall, P.A. (1990) Cultural differences on perceived quality of life. *Seminars in Oncology Nursing*, 6(4): 278–84.

Mathiesen, C.M. and Stam, H.J. (1995) Renegotiating identity: cancer narratives. *Sociology of Health and Illness*, 17(3): 283–306.

Mattingly, C. (1994) The concept of therapeutic emplotment. *Social Science and Medicine*, 38(6): 811–22.

Mechanic, D. (1992) Sociological research in health and the American sociopolitical context: the changing fortunes of medical sociology. *Social Science and Medicine*, 36(2): 95–102.

Mechanic, D. (1995) Emerging trends in the application of the social services to health and medicine. *Social Science and Medicine*, 40(11): 1491–6.

Meredith, P. (1993) Patient satisfaction in decision-making and consent to treatment: the case of general surgery. *Sociology of Health and Illness*, 15(3): 315–36.

Meyerowitz, B.E. (1993) Quality of life in breast cancer patients: the contribution of data to the care of patients. *European Journal of Cancer*, 29a (Suppl. 1): 559–62.

Millar, B. (1997) The stakes are high. *Health Service Journal*, 24 April: 1–2.

Mishler, E.G. (1986) *Research Interviewing: Context and Narrative*. Cambridge MA: Harvard University Press.

Mohan, J. (1991) Privatization in the British health sector: a challenge to the NHS?, in J. Gabe, M. Calnan and M. Bury (eds) *The Sociology of the Health Service*. London: Routledge.

Moinpour, C.M., Feigl, P., Metch, B., Hayden, K.A., Meyskens, F.L. and Crowley, J. (1989) Quality of life end points in cancer clinical trials: review and recommendations. *Journal of the National Cancer Institute*, 81(7): 485–95.

Montazeri, A., McEwen, J. and Gillis, C.R. (1996) Quality of life in patients with ovarian cancer. Current state of research. *Supportive Care in Cancer*, 4: 169–79.

Moore, A. (1997) All pulling together. *Health Service Journal*, 24 April: 8–9.

Morris, T., Blake, S. and Buckley, M. (1985) Development of a method for rating cognitive responses to a diagnosis of cancer. *Social Science and Medicine*, 20(8): 795–802.

Morris, T., Greer, H.S. and White, P. (1977) Psychological and social adjustment to mastectomy. *Cancer*, 40: 2381–7.

Morse, J.M. and Johnson, J.L. (eds) (1991) *The Illness Experience: Dimensions of Suffering*. Newbury Park: Sage.

Moynihan, C. (1987) Testicular cancer: the psychosocial problems of patients and their relations. *Cancer Surveys*, 6(3): 477–510.

Moynihan, C. (1991) Testicular cancer, in M. Watson (ed.) *Cancer Patient Care: Psychosocial Treatment Methods*. Cambridge: Cambridge University Press.

Nagpal, R. and Sell, H. (1985) Subjective wellbeing, in *SEARO Regional Health Papers, 7.* New Delhi: World Health Organization.

Nerenz, D.R. and Levanthal, H. (1983) Self-regulation theory in chronic illness, in T.G. Burish and L.A. Bradley (eds) *Coping with Chronic Disease: Research and Applications.* New York: Academic Press.

Nordin, K., Glimelius, B., Påhlman, L. and Sjoden, P. (1996) Anxiety, depression and worry in gastrointestinal cancer patients attending medical follow-up control visits. *Acta Oncologica,* 35(4): 411–16.

O'Boyle, C.A. (1994) The schedule for the evaluation of individual quality of life. *International Journal of Mental Health,* 23: 3–23.

O'Boyle, C.A. and Waldron, D. (1997) Quality of life issues in palliative medicine. *Neurology,* 244 (Suppl. 4): S18–S25.

Olweny, C.L.M., Juttner, C.A., Rofe, P., Barrow, G., Esterman, A., Waltham, R. et al. (1993) Long term effects of cancer treatment and consequences of cure: cancer survivors enjoy quality of life similar to their neighbours. *European Journal of Cancer,* 29a (Suppl. 6): 826–30.

Patrick, D.L. and Erickson, P. (1988) Assessing health-related quality of life for clinical decision-making, in S.R. Walker and R.M. Rosser (eds) *Quality of Life: Assessment and Application.* London: MTP Press Ltd.

Pietroni, P. (1990) *The Greening of Medicine.* London: Gollancz.

Pope, C. (1991) Trouble in store: some thoughts on the management of waiting lists. *Sociology of Health and Illness,* 13: 194–221.

Potter, J. and Wetherell, M. (1987) *Discourse and Social Psychology: Beyond Attitudes and Behaviour.* London: Sage.

Rappaport, H. (1990) *Marking Time.* New York: Simon and Schuster.

Richards, M.A. (1997) Calman-Hine: two years on. *Palliative Medicine,* 11: 433–4.

Rineberg, B.A. (1991) Health care rationing: a quality of life issue. *Orthopedics,* 14(7): 815.

Ritchie, S. (1992) A declaration of rights for people with cancer. *Journal of Cancer Care,* 1: 69–72.

Rodrigue, J.R., Behen, J.M. and Tumlin, T. (1994) Multidimensional determinants of psychological adjustment to cancer. *Psycho-Oncology,* 3: 205–14.

Rosser, R. (1993) The history of health-related quality of life in $10^{1/2}$ paragraphs. *Journal of the Royal Society of Medicine,* 86(6): 315–18.

Sacks, H. (1989) Lecture 5, in G. Jefferson (ed.), *Lectures 1964–1965. Human Studies,* 12(3/4): 211–15.

Sandelowski, M. and Corson Jones, L. (1996) 'Healing fictions': stories of choosing in the aftermath of the detection of fetal abnormalities. *Social Science and Medicine,* 42(3): 353–61.

Saunders, C. (1989) *Living with Dying: The Management of Terminal Disease,* 2nd edn. Oxford: Oxford University Press.

Schipper, H. (1990) Principles of the clinical paradigm. *Journal of Psychosocial Oncology,* 8(2–3): 171–85.

Schipper, H., Clinch, J., McMurray, A. and Levitt, M. (1984) Measuring the quality of life of cancer patients: the functional living index – cancer: development and validation. *Journal of Clinical Oncology,* 2: 472–83.

Schutz, A. and Luckman, T. (1974) *The Structures of the Lifeworld.* London: Heinemann.

Seiden Miller, R. (1978) The social construction and reconstruction of physiological events: acquiring the pregnancy identity, in N.K. Denzin (ed.) *Studies in Symbolic Interaction: An Annual Compilation of Research*, vol. 1. Greenwich, CN: JAI Press Inc.

Selby, P., Chapman, J.A.W., Etazadi-Amoli, J. *et al.* (1984) The development of a method for assessing the quality of life of cancer patients. *British Journal of Cancer*, 50: 13–22.

Selby, P. and Robertson, B. (1986) Measurement of quality of life in patients with cancer. *Cancer Surveys*, 6(3): 521–43.

Sharma, U.M. (1990) Using alternative therapies: marginal medicine and central concerns, in P. Abbott and G. Payne (eds) *New Directions in the Sociology of Health*, Explorations in Sociology No. 36. London: Falmer Press.

Sigurdardottir, V., Bolund, C. and Sullivan, M. (1996) Quality of life evaluation by the EORTC questionnaire technique in patients with generalized malignant melanoma on chemotherapy. *Acta Oncologica*, 35(2): 149–58.

Sikora, K. (1997) Wheels within wheels. *Health Service Journal*, 24 April: 12.

Silberfarb, P.M., Maurer, L.H. and Crouthamel, C.S. (1980) Psychosocial aspects of neoplastic disease: I. Functional status of breast cancer patients during different treatment regimens. *American Journal of Psychiatry*, 137(4): 450–5.

Silverman, D. (1985) *Qualitative Methodology and Sociology: Describing the Social World*. Vermont: Gower Publishing Company.

Silverman, D. and Perakyla, A. (1990) AIDS counselling: the interactional organisation of talk about 'delicate' issues. *Sociology of Health and Illness*, 12(3): 293–318.

Simiroff, L.A. and Fetting, J.H. (1991) Factors affecting treatment decisions for a life-threatening illness: the case of medical treatment of breast cancer. *Social Science and Medicine*, 32(7): 813–18.

Somerfield, M. and Curbow, B. (1992) Methodological issues and research strategies in the study of coping with cancer. *Social Science and Medicine*, 34(11): 1203–16.

Spicer, J. and Chamberlain, K. (1996) Developing psychosocial theory in health psychology: problems and prospects. *Journal of Health Psychology*, 1(2): 161–71.

Spiegel, D. (1997) Psychosocial aspects of breast cancer treatment. *Seminars in Oncology*, 24(1)(Suppl. 1): S1.36–S1.47.

Spitzer, N.O., Dobson, A.J., Hall, J., Chesterman, E., Levi, J., Shepherd, R. *et al.* (1981) Measuring the quality of life in cancer patients. *Journal of Chronic Disease*, 34: 585–97.

Stainton-Rogers, W. (1991) *Explaining Health and Illness: An Exploration of Diversity*. London: Harvester Wheatsheaf.

Strauss, A.L. and Corbin, J. (1990) *Basics of Qualitative Research: Grounded Theory Procedures and Techniques*, 2nd edn. Newbury Park: Sage.

Strauss, A.L. and Corbin, J. (1994) Grounded theory methodology: an overview, in N.K. Denzin and Y.S. Lincoln (eds) *Handbook of Qualitative Research*. Thousand Oaks, CA: Sage.

Strauss, A. and Glaser, B.G. (1975) *Chronic Illness and the Quality of Life*. St Louis: C.V. Mosby.

Strauss, A., Fagerhaugh, S., Suczek, B. and Wiener, C. (1985) *Social Organization of Medical Work*. Chicago: University of Chicago Press.

Temoshok, L. and Heller, B.W. (1984) On comparing apples, oranges and fruit salad: a methodological overview of medical outcomes studies in psychosocial oncology, in C.L. Cooper (ed.) *Psychosocial Stress and Cancer*. New York: John Wiley and Sons.

Townsend, P., Davidson, N. and Whitehead, M. (1988) *Inequalities in Health*. London: Penguin.

Traynor, B.M. (1992) Quality of life. *Journal of Cancer Care*, 1: 35–40.

Turner, B.S. (1995) *Medical Power and Social Knowledge*, 2nd edn. London: Sage.

Van der Waal, M.A.E., Casparie, A.F. and Lako, C.J. (1996) Quality of care: a comparison of preferences between medical specialists and patients with chronic diseases. *Social Science and Medicine*, 42(5): 643–9.

Van Knippenberg, F.C.E., Out, J.J., Tilanus, H.W., Mud, H.J., Hop, W.L.J. and Verhage, F. (1992) Quality of life in patients with resected oesophageal cancer. *Social Science and Medicine*, 35(2): 139–45.

Watson, M. and Morris, T. (eds) (1985) *Psychological Aspects of Cancer*. Oxford: Pergamon Press.

Weisman, A.D., Worden, J.W. and Sobel, H.J. (1980) 'Psychosocial screening and intervention with cancer patients', Research Report, *Project Omega*. Department of Psychiatry, Harvard Medical School.

Wellisch, D., Landsverk, J., Guidera, K., Pasnan, R. and Fawzy, F. (1983) Evaluation of psychosocial problems of the homebound cancer patient: I: methodology and problem frequencies. *Psychosomatic Medicine*, 45: 11–21.

Whitehead, M. (1988) *The Health Divide*. London: Penguin.

Whynes, D.K. (1992) Health economics and cancer care. *Journal of Cancer Care*, 1: 131–7.

Williams, G.H. (1991) Disablement and the ideological crisis in health care. *Social Science and Medicine*, 32(4): 517–24.

Williams, O.A. (1993) Patient knowledge of operative care. *Journal of the Royal Society of Medicine*, 86(6): 328–31.

Williams, R. (1989) Awareness and control of dying: some paradoxical trends in public opinion. *Sociology of Health and Illness*, 11(3): 201–12.

Yoshida, K.K. (1993) Reshaping of self: a pendular reconstruction of self and identity among adults with traumatic spinal chord injury. *Sociology of Health and Illness*, 15(2): 217–45.

Zigmond, A.S. and Snaith, R.P. (1983) The hospital anxiety and depression scale. *ACTA Psychiatrica Scandinavia*, 67: 361–70.

Index

NEW THEMES IN PALLIATIVE CARE

David Clark, Jo Hockley and Sam Ahmedzai (eds)

Palliative care is moving through an important period of expansion and development, spreading beyond its original hospice base to encompass care in the community, in hospitals, health centres, clinics and nursing homes. It can now be found in over 70 countries of the world. What challenges does this multidisciplinary speciality face as it seeks to combine high grade pain and symptom control with sensitive psychological, spiritual and social care? What are the implications of current constraints on health policy and planning? How do ethical issues about resource allocation and end of life care impinge? Can palliative care be further extended to include conditions other than cancer?

New Themes in Palliative Care addresses these and many related issues in ways which will be readily accessible to students of health and social care as well as to those involved in purchasing or providing palliative care services, and to social scientists interested in chronic illness, death and dying. Its editors are respected experts in the field with backgrounds in the social sciences, nursing and medicine and the book's contributors include leading international figures from a wide range of palliative care and academic disciplines.

Contents
Introduction – Part 1: Policy, ethics, evidence – Introduction to Part 1 – Assessing needs and effectiveness: is palliative care a special case? – Costs of palliative care – Resource allocation and palliative care – Half full or half empty? The impact of health reforms on palliative care services in the UK – Part 2: Service developments – Introduction to Part 2 – The evolution of the hospice approach – Terminal care in South Australia: historical aspects and equity issues – Palliative care in India – Palliative home care – A Swedish model of home care – Rational planning and policy implementation in palliative care – Palliative care in eastern Europe – Is hospice a western concept? A personal view of palliative care in Asia – The WHO cancer pain and palliative care programme – Part 3: Clinical issues – Introduction to Part 3 – Therapeutic innovations – Beyond cancer? – Teamwork in end-of-life care: a nurse-physician perspective on introducing physicians to palliative care concepts – Voluntary euthanasia in terminal illness – New approaches to care – Index.

Contributors
Barbro Beck-Friis, Kenneth Boyd, Gilly Burn, David Clark, Jessica Corner, Nessa Coyle, Carol David, Georgio Di Mola, Robert Dunlop, Calliope Farsides, M. Dulce Fontanals, Eve Garrard, Rob George, Xavier Gómez-Batiste, Pauline Heather, Jo Hockley, Roger W. Hunt, Jane M. Ingham, Jacek Łuczak, Ian Maddocks, Karen Mallett, Helen Malson, Francesc Martinez, Brenda Neale, David Oxenham, Margaret Robbins, Jordi Roca, Pere Roige-Canals, Frances Sheldon, Neil Small, Jan Stjernsward, Jo Sykes, Elisabeth Valles, David Whynes.

320pp   0 335 19605 5 (Paperback)   0 335 19606 3 (Hardback)